PRAISE FOR

Healing Multiple Sclerosis

"A woman who's done something really incredible. . . . I want
people to go out and get a copy of the book."
—MONTEL WILLIAMS on *The Montel Williams Show*

"*Healing Multiple Sclerosis* not only reveals a new paradigm
underlying this disease but provides a powerful user-friendly
therapeutic approach. This is a vitally important must read for
patients and families alike."
—DAVID PERLMUTTER, MD, FACN, author of
The Better Brain Book and *Power Up Your Brain*

"*Healing Multiple Sclerosis* is a must-read book for those
with multiple sclerosis. There is so much you can do to
begin restoring your health and vitality without resorting to
expensive, toxic prescription medications."
—TERRY WAHLS, MD, author of *Minding My
Mitochondria: How I Overcame Secondary Progressive
Multiple Sclerosis and Got Out of My Wheelchair*

"A book filled with useful information that, when combined
with the desire and intention of someone who chooses to be
a survivor and participate in their healing, can provide results
which far surpass what is expected."
—BERNIE SIEGEL, MD, *New York Times* best-selling
author of *Love, Medicine & Miracles* and *Help Me
to Heal*

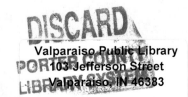

"Ann Boroch's book is right on the mark! . . . Provides workable, natural solutions for a practical self-help program that anybody with a desire to get well can follow. Written in four parts, consisting of her personal journey, the causes of MS, and the solutions, Ms. Boroch's book also provides a wonderful treatment section chock-full of user-friendly charts, supplementation programs, recipes, and resources. Ann Boroch will inspire and enlighten you. By following her program, you will not only experience more energy, heightened vitality, and mental clarity, but your overall health is sure to improve."

> —ANN LOUISE GITTLEMAN, PHD, CNS, *New York Times* best-selling author of 30 books on health and healing

New Revised Edition

HEALING MULTIPLE SCLEROSIS

Diet, Detox & Nutritional Makeover for Total Recovery

~~~~~~

ANN BOROCH, CNC

Foreword by Ann Louise Gittleman, PhD, CNS

QUINTESSENTIAL HEALING PUBLISHING

For information, contact:

Quintessential Healing Publishing, Inc.
11712 Moorpark St., Suite 106
Studio City, CA 91604

Website: www.annboroch.com
Email: ann@annboroch.com
Phone: 818.763.8282

For foreign and translation rights, contact Nigel J. Yorwerth
Email: nigel@publishingcoaches.com

Library of Congress Control Number: 2013930100

ISBN: 978-0-9773446-4-2 (paperback)
ISBN: 978-0-9773446-5-9 (ebook)

10 9 8 7 6 5 4 3 2

Cover design: Geyrhalter & Company and Allison Boroch, Designing Elements

Interior design and production: Robert S. Tinnon Design and Becky Sheehan

This book is intended to serve only as a resource and educational guide. I cannot assume medical or legal responsibility for having the contents of this book considered as a prescription for anyone. Treatment of health disorders needs to be supervised by your physician or licensed health-care professional.

To my mother,
you are my Rock of Gibraltar . . .
and to those heroes
who have the courage and tenacity
to conquer disease

CONTENTS

FOREWORD

True healing is like peeling the skin of an onion. There is no one single cause, and the various layers differ with each individual.

As the author of twenty-five books on health and healing, I believe with all my heart and all my soul that there is an answer to every disease—we simply have to look in the right place. The body is an incredible system with an infinite capacity to heal, provided that we lessen our toxic load and provide the right nourishment and environment for regeneration to occur.

The sad news is that today we are living in a sea of toxins that are making us fat and making us sick. For the first time in history, cancer overtook heart disease as the number-one killer of all Americans in 2004.

According to the National Cancer Institute, there are over 100,000 chemicals used by Americans in household cleaners, solvents, pesticides, food additives, lawn care, and other products. And every year, another 1,000 are introduced. One new chemical enters industrial use every twenty minutes. The average person living in twenty-first-century America is now contaminated with up to 500 industrial toxins, the majority of which haven't been tested for harmful effects. The CDC has been keeping an eye out on our collective "body burden" for a while and has found that we are all 100 percent polluted.

Over the past sixty years, our diets, lifestyles, and environment have undergone a revolution, placing a huge burden on our body's detoxification organs. Our tired and overloaded livers are being exposed to more toxins than they can handle; our

GI tracts are sluggish and constipated without enough fiber-rich food; we are lacking critical nutrients needed for the liver's detox pathways; and the liver's detox enzymes are being inhibited by common medications, excess sugar, caffeine, and trans fats.

Cancer rates have risen between 20 and 50 percent since 1970. Breast cancer will impact one out of eight American women if we live long enough. Asthma has increased by 75 percent since 1980. The diagnosis of autism has increased nearly 20 percent every year. Type 2 diabetes is epidemic among young people in their thirties, while the incidence of autoimmune diseases like lupus, rheumatoid arthritis, and multiple sclerosis has gone through the roof.

And so I am very pleased to say that Ann Boroch's book is right on the mark!

Her tumultuous four-year journey of reversing multiple sclerosis taught her firsthand to examine the layers that the body and mind take on to create disease. The result of her journey is a landmark book that identifies and unifies seemingly unrelated "root" causes that go beyond petrochemicals—and that targets candida/fungus, diet, silver fillings, parasites, vaccinations, geopathic stresses, trauma, and genetics, which are underlying hidden factors present in almost all autoimmune diseases. Best of all, Ms. Boroch provides workable natural solutions for a practical self-help program that anybody with a desire to get well can follow.

Written in four parts, consisting of her personal journey, the causes of MS, and the solutions, Ms. Boroch's book also provides a wonderful treatment section chock-full of user-friendly charts, supplementation programs, recipes, and resources.

Ann Boroch will inspire and enlighten you. By following her program, you will not only experience more energy, heightened vitality, and mental clarity, but your overall health is sure to improve. Ms. Boroch is to be congratulated for her courage and knowledge that disease is a wake-up call to clean up your act from the inside out!

ANN LOUISE GITTLEMAN, PhD, CNS

New York Times best-selling author of
The Fat Flush Plan, Before the Change, and
The Fast Track One-Day Detox Diet

PREFACE

My doctor leafed through page after page of my medical chart—EEG results, neurological exams, evoked potential tests. . . . I had undergone two weeks of tests hoping to learn what was causing the spasms, numbness, tingling, and other neurological symptoms that had left me barely able to walk on my own. "Well, Ann," he said, "the good news is, you don't have cancer. The bad news is . . . you have multiple sclerosis." With those words, I became a statistic, one of an estimated three million people worldwide—500,000 in the United States alone—who are afflicted by the debilitating disease of multiple sclerosis.

". . . incurable . . . experiment with chemotherapy . . . slow the inevitable deterioration. . . ."

He went on speaking, but I was in such shock that his words made no sense to me. Traditional Western medicine had failed to cure me of serious mononucleosis five years earlier. I had no confidence that it could help me now.

I left his office, and after two weeks of physical suffering, mental turmoil, and emotional torture, I turned my back on the traditional medical treatments for MS. I was only twenty-four, and terrified, but I refused to accept the prospect of spending my life in a wheelchair. "I will not be another MS statistic," I promised myself. And slowly, bit by bit, I created my own self-care program based on integrative medicine methods.

Four tumultuous years later, I reversed MS.

You must understand that health is more than just the physical body. Health means a balance of the body, mind, emotions, and spirit. When you experience a chronic disease, all facets of the self must be examined. This means moving beyond the symptoms to address diet, lifestyle, stress, exercise, negative thoughts, fear-based emotions, and self-limiting belief systems.

Eventually, I hope, the usual paradigm in Western medicine will shift to a realization that even if two people have the same disease, they must be treated as individuals based on the knowledge that each person's history is unique, that health is more than just treating the physical body, and that it is essential to go to the root cause. Then cures will be the rule, not the exception to the rule.

Most important, health is a choice. Yes, the body has an innate inner intelligence that works at keeping itself balanced through the process known as homeostasis. But this is not enough to maintain health if you are making unhealthy choices, entertaining negative thoughts, bombarding your body with depleted foods, overwhelming it with stress, and holding on to fear-based emotions. Whenever you make the apparently simple choice of what to eat each day, you are actually choosing whether you want health—or not.

Even as I took the first steps on my healing journey, it was clear to me that I would be moving not only toward achieving recovery, but also toward helping others to move through the complexities of autoimmune disease. Today I am a nutritionist and naturopath with a fifteen-year practice, during which I've seen thousands of clients for various health conditions. Based on both my personal and my professional experience, it is my responsibility, and my passion, not just to educate you about the causes of MS and how to reverse it, but also to inspire you with the knowledge that you can triumph.

Society, your family, and your peers have more or less conditioned you to believe that you are powerless when it comes to MS—that drugs are your only option for living with this diagnosis. That is not so. There is a hidden truth to healing that has always been with us. This truth is the incredible individual power you possess to transform yourself—your body, your spirit, your mind, and your emotions. Making a choice to become healthy and then backing it up with belief and conviction are the keys to coming into your own power and turning around any disease.

This book is presented in four sections:

- Part One, "My Healing Journey," recounts my personal transformational journey and how I cured MS.

- Part Two, "The Real Cause of Multiple Sclerosis," describes all the causes of MS.

- Part Three, "You Can Heal Yourself: The Solutions," explains the solutions and why they are effective.

- Part Four, "Your Treatment Plan," gives you user-friendly charts, recipes, and exercises so you can create your own self-help treatment program.

ACKNOWLEDGMENTS

This book is the product of much time, reworking, and editing, and I'm grateful to everyone who has helped me to shape it:

- Monica Faulkner, thank you for making my vision of this book become a reality.
- Fabian Geyrhalter and Allison Boroch, thank you for your creativity with the cover.
- Patricia Spadaro and Janet Chaikin, for your quintessential editing.
- Nigel Yorwerth, for your guidance in helping shape, package, and market this book and for serving as my foreign rights agent.

As is true for us all, my journey has been blessed with much support and guidance along the way. I want to express my sincere gratitude to

- All my friends, teachers, and health-care professionals who have helped me reach this point.
- My clients, who have taught me to be the best I can be.
- The late Dr. William Crook, who was a model of courage in writing his truth and helping so many.
- Dr. Bob Drosman, you are a shining light—thank you for being there and supporting my healing journey.

- The late Peter Ulikhanov, a great healer and mentor who gave me the confidence to be the successful healer that I am.

- Julie Jones-Ufkes, Alison Moon, and Andrea Berman, for your recipe contributions.

- Linda Jeckel and Perry Desiante (Pa), for helping me during my darkest days.

- Josh Willow, Irene Zaragoza, and Liz Lachman for your loyal friendship and support.

- Mom, you're my biggest cheerleader and have always been there for me.

- Jasmine Contor, because without you, there was no hope or light at the end of the tunnel. I am eternally grateful for you and your magnificent gift.

PART ONE

MY
HEALING
JOURNEY

CHAPTER ONE

CONQUERING MULTIPLE SCLEROSIS

As you will discover by reading my story, there are many ways to break down a body and create disease. I have learned that those components are not purely physical. When it comes to autoimmune disease, the imbalances of emotional, mental, and spiritual stress are just as important as poor diet, environmental toxins, and genetics.

My story is tumultuous, but it does not mean that everyone with multiple sclerosis (MS) must go through the depths and layers as I did. What is important about my journey is that I now have the passion and knowledge to educate others. In this book I will reveal the causes of MS and the solutions available to you to heal it.

Let me take you back to where it all began . . .

～～～

I'd like to say I grew up in a happy, picture-perfect "Father Knows Best" household with mommy and daddy, but I didn't. My parents met and married at a very young age. I was conceived in a Corvette on the back roads of a small Connecticut town. Shortly thereafter, they moved to Southern California and settled in Montclair, where I was born in 1965. I grew up an only child. My mother is a beautiful, strong Italian woman with a great sense of humor. My father is a gregarious businessman of German-Polish descent. They made a handsome couple, but bliss was short-lived and they divorced when I was three.

As a teenager, I looked back at old pictures and felt a sense of loss and wondered what it would have been like to grow up with both parents. Instead, I lived with my mother and saw my father every other weekend. Each household was a different environment, and I found solace in each for what the other one couldn't offer. I was the center of attention in each home until the age of nine, when my father remarried and had my only half brother.

The rivalry between my parents started early on in my life, and so did my anxiety. Their divorce was bitter and I felt their anger towards each other throughout my childhood. As a way of distracting myself, I started to participate in a variety of sports. My mother provided the funds for me to learn horseback riding, ice-skating, soccer, basketball, and baseball. As good as I was, I ended up getting injured in every sport I played and started to become filled with doubt and fear when it came to playing any sport. In retrospect, I realize that my fears and doubts were contributing to a vicious cycle of injury.

Besides these injuries, illness in my life was almost as commonplace as breathing. My childhood was centered around visiting doctors' offices for colds, ear and sinus infections, the flu, and impetigo—so frequently that I developed an immunity to penicillin by the age of nine. I had no idea that the standard routine of taking antibiotics would eventually send my body cascading in a downward spiral.

And little did I know that my poor eating habits of consuming sugar and processed foods were paving the way to constant illness. The sugar I ate contributed to rotting almost every tooth I had. As a sugarholic, I had an entire mouthful of silver-mercury fillings by the age of twelve. With each dentist visit and each filling, I became less afraid of going because I knew it was just a way to stop the toothache so I could eat more candy.

I grew up feeling like a mental and emotional Ping-Pong ball, caught in the dynamics of a dysfunctional family and constantly being batted back and forth between my parents, with only my grandparents as buffers. On the outside I seemed to have it all under control. I was doing well in school, I had friends, and I had learned to appease whichever parent I was with. But inside I was battling to find safe ground.

COPING

The dynamics between my mother and me were intense. It was a love-hate relationship. She was, and still is, loving, spontaneous, fun, and full of energy. She was also controlling, critical, and strict, with a fiery Italian temper. Our Italian household meant shoes and spoons came flying my way if I didn't behave. I feared her temper and felt my every action was scrutinized. There isn't a time that I can remember feeling accepted for just being me. I became obsessed with being perfect, but the harder I tried to be perfect in her eyes, the clumsier I became and the more stupid I felt.

My father was an alcoholic and emotionally detached. His preoccupation with business left little room for me. More than anything, I wanted to be "daddy's little girl," but to no avail. My father didn't know how to reach out emotionally and our connection was superficial. The end result was that I feared and mistrusted the man whose love and validation I so yearned for.

The psychological and emotional events that took place throughout my childhood were setting the stage for illness.

Fear-based emotions surrounding my abandonment issues, such as guilt, fear, and anger, were settling into my body's cellular memory. Unconsciously, I was adopting a pattern of getting sick or injuring myself to receive unconditional love. That was how I coped.

To make matters worse, I developed an addiction to comfort foods and lived on excessive amounts of sugar, refined carbohydrates, sodas, and processed foods. My paternal grandmother was very influential in my life. Her unconditional love neutralized some of my stress. She had a heart of gold and loved to spoil me with her delicious cooking. Though she cooked everything from scratch, I ate a lot of sugar and refined carbs from all the homemade pies, cakes, and cookies she made. Sugar became my vice to pacify my emotions.

At that time, I didn't know how detrimental refined sugars were and that they weaken the immune system by stripping essential vitamins and minerals needed to run the body. Also, sugar makes the body acidic and increases inflammation, which lays the perfect breeding ground for disease to start. I was trying to kill my emotional pain, but in reality I was depleting my immune system.

SPIRALING DOWN

At age nineteen, on a beautiful Sunday afternoon in April, I went to the mall with a couple of friends. I walked into a candy store and suddenly everything went into slow motion. My skin felt numb, my head felt heavy and cloudy, and I couldn't feel the ground under my feet. A wave of panic overcame me, yet no one noticed. A hot flash swept over me as I stumbled from the store to shake off this feeling. I asked my friends to take me home because I didn't feel well. They thought I just needed to get some food in my system. I got home, ate a little something, and went to bed early.

I awoke the next morning to the thought that the previous day had just been a nightmare and I would be back to normal. But as I opened my eyes I felt an enormous heaviness in my head. I sat up and felt disoriented. The symptoms from the day before had intensified. I skipped school and went to the doctor. After examining me and drawing blood for tests, which came back negative, he told me I had a viral infection in my chest and sent me home with antibiotics.

My symptoms never left, and a month later my condition had worsened. I went through another round of tests and found out that I had mononucleosis and Epstein-Barr virus. My symptoms were fatigue, disorientation, brain fog, allergies (dietary and environmental), chest constriction, ear and sinus pain and pressure, sore throat, constipation, weight loss, depression, and dizziness. For two months I was exhausted and lay in bed with no signs of improvement. I went to several specialists searching for an answer. Over the next eight months I saw seven specialists, who prescribed more than twenty different medications, mostly antibiotics and steroids. I took every test imaginable—MRIs, EKGs, hearing tests, urine samples—and everything came up negative.

My whole world had been shaken to the core. I began feeling anger and frustration toward my doctors and traditional medicine for prescribing drug after drug that offered no signs of relief. More systems were breaking down in my body as a result of all the medication. Because doctors didn't examine or talk about lifestyle habits such as poor diet and stress in connection with illness, it made it even more difficult to uncover the root cause of what was ailing me. Lastly, I had no specific religion to lean on and I felt lost and hopeless. For the first time in my life I wanted to die.

MY SEARCH TO GET WELL

One day near the end of November, my mother went to lunch with a friend. When he asked how I was feeling, she said I was getting worse. He told her about a woman friend of his who was a medical intuitive.

My condition had worsened to such a degree that my mother was willing to try anything, so she contacted the medical intuitive, and within a week I received a detailed written reading in the mail. She said I had a severe condition called *candidiasis*, an overgrowth of the yeast *Candida albicans*, brought about by a lifetime of antibiotic overuse, steroids, and a poor diet consisting mainly of refined sugars and carbohydrates. The yeast toxins had moved from my gastrointestinal tract into my bloodstream and activated an antibody reaction, which in turn triggered an excessive production of white blood cells, causing symptoms similar to mononucleosis.

She also said that when my attacks were extreme, borderline symptoms of leukemia appeared. I was also suffering from a breakdown in red blood cell production, as well as dietary deficiencies and an inability to synthesize amino acids. The most critical factor was for me to regulate my diet by eliminating refined sugars, processed foods, dairy products, and yeast-containing foods (peanuts, breads, mushrooms, vinegars, and most condiments) and to take an antifungal medication to eradicate the yeast overgrowth.

A week after receiving the medical intuitive's diagnosis, I came across a newly released book by William Crook, MD, an emeritus member of the American Academy of Pediatrics and the American College of Allergy, Asthma, and Immunology. It was called *The Yeast Connection: A Medical Breakthrough,*[1] and it confirmed my condition. I learned that candidiasis is a silent epidemic in the United States because of our poor diets and overuse of antibiotics and steroids.

Candida albicans is a single-celled yeast that naturally lives in our intestinal tracts, on our mucous membranes, and on our skin. Dr. Crook explained that taking antibiotics wipes out both the good and bad bacteria in our bodies, but doesn't kill the yeast. The absence of good bacteria allows the yeast to continually thrive on a poor diet of refined sugars, dairy, alcohol, and fermented foods. We then end up craving more of the foods that keep the yeast multiplying.

Over time, the yeast turns into a fungus that migrates through the intestinal walls and into the bloodstream. To make matters worse, the yeast produce seventy-nine by-products that weaken the immune system and create more imbalances. Once in the bloodstream, the yeast and its by-products can attack the genetically weakest and most vulnerable systems in the body. The brain fog I was experiencing was from one of the main by-products, acetaldehyde, which breaks down into ethyl alcohol in the liver and was causing me to feel disoriented and throwing off my coordination as if I were drunk.

Most important, Dr. Crook explained that yeast/fungal overgrowth will not go away and allow the body to return to its normal state unless a person is treated with an antifungal drug and makes dietary modifications. When I read his book, I actually cried for joy. I felt relieved knowing that I was being guided on the right track. At last I was finding concrete answers. The correlations were easy. I was a classic case, given my history of an extremely poor diet and the countless times I was prescribed antibiotics and steroids. Even while I was reading the book, I was taking yet another round of antibiotics.

The intuitive's reading and Dr. Crook's book instructed me to start taking Nystatin, an antifungal drug. Nystatin is a concentrated soil-based organism and is listed in the *Physician's Desk Reference* as one of the least toxic drugs and as safe for pregnant women and infants. I was also instructed to change my diet. Refined sugar was lethal to my body and I needed to avoid any form of it—dextrose, fructose, maple syrup, molasses, and brown sugar. I was also advised to avoid dairy, wheat, refined carbohydrates, alcohol, and fermented products.

I began to eat foods I hadn't even known existed, such as millet and quinoa. I drank water on a regular basis for the first time. I had grown up thinking the whole world of food consisted of pasta, canned soups, frozen dinners, sodas, and Ding Dongs. This was a rude awakening!

After one year of following this program I returned to health and vitality. I was amazed and hungry for knowledge that would expand my own empowerment. I wanted to know what my health challenges were trying to "tell" me. I started to read and do research on how the body and mind worked together. Yet as time went on, my old patterns of consuming sugar and feeling stressed resurfaced.

MS DIAGNOSIS

Four years later, at age twenty-four, my life again came to a screeching halt. I was eating at a restaurant with my friend Linda when I was slammed with an attack. I couldn't move, speak, or swallow. Panic surged through my mind and body. I gasped for air as my body spasmed uncontrollably. It lasted for only thirty seconds, but it felt much longer.

After the attack subsided I asked her to take me home. She had to help carry me out to the car because I was still having spasms. Linda called my mother, who came to my rescue immediately and stayed with me late into the night, covering me in blankets and trying to calm me. I couldn't stop the shaking, which seemed to be coming from the deepest parts of me, and my thoughts were fragmented. I knew this was serious. Finally, no longer able to fight the fatigue, I fell asleep.

The next day my mother took me to a specialist. I had extreme muscle weakness and fatigue and was barely able to walk into his office. Some parts of my body felt numb and I was having trouble speaking. I loathed being in a doctor's office again, but I was too unstable to think of an alternative. He did a complete neurological examination and sent me off to the hospital to take a number of tests, including an EEG (electroencephalogram, which measures brain waves) and EPs (evoked potentials, which record the nervous system's electrical responses to the stimulation of specific sensory pathways, such as visual, auditory, and general sensory).

For the next several days my body remained incapacitated. My mind was reeling with fear-filled emotions and thoughts. When I entered the doctor's office to get the results, I was trembling.

He sat me and my mother down and opened my chart. "Well, the good news is, you don't have cancer. The bad news is you have multiple sclerosis."

I was speechless. Now that I finally had a diagnosis and knew what was wrong with me, I didn't know whether I felt relief or terror. The last words I remember him saying were "Multiple sclerosis . . . incurable, but there are experimental drugs like chemotherapy to work with. . . ."

My mother, offended by the doctor's insensitive manner, helped me hobble out of the office. I was devastated and cried all the way home. I felt my life was over. I was only twenty-four, but so physically ravaged that I couldn't bear to think about my future. How would I ever begin to accept this diagnosis and move on with what was left of my life?

I couldn't.

I had to quit work and struggled each day just to exist. The first year was unbearable. The days droned on with endless symptoms, constantly reminding me that my body had completely changed again. My symptoms continued to worsen, giving me no periods of rest. For the first few months I was bedridden. Because MS is an autoimmune disease of the central nervous system, I had daily immune-response attacks in which I would lose control over my motor skills. My body would spasm and tremor uncontrollably. I was unable to carry out coordinated movements such as walking. I experienced numbness and tingling in my limbs, muscle weakness, impaired sensory perception, convulsive tremors, bladder dysfunction, and nervous exhaustion. My ability to speak, chew, and swallow was impaired. I also had trouble formulating thoughts and accessing memory.

The essence of life that I had taken for granted was now gone. Everything had happened so fast. I felt like someone who had been incarcerated for ten years, then released just long enough to adjust, only to be suddenly thrown right back in. I spent many days lying on the floor completely terrorized by a body that wouldn't function. I cried for hours and became exhausted from obsessing and trying to tolerate the bizarre symptoms I was experiencing. Every part of my body felt completely exhausted. My central nervous system, which controls everything in the body, was completely incapacitated. I now knew what it felt like to be a quadriplegic. The utter horror of having no movement was enough to drive me insane. I lived in constant fear that my next breath would be my last.

I finally decided to call the medical intuitive I had previously contacted to ask for another reading. Within a couple of days, I had a phone consultation with her. When she confirmed that I did indeed have MS, my breath stopped and my heart sank.

But before I could react, she added, "You have the power to eradicate this disease."

"How?"

She told me to get back on Nystatin, to clean up my diet once again by staying away from sugars, yeast, dairy products, and alcohol. She also said I needed to have my fifteen silver-mercury fillings removed.

"Finally, it's essential for you to believe—to know—that you can eradicate this so-called incurable disease," she said.

When I hung up the phone, part of me felt positive and hopeful, but another part of me felt clouded with more questions and uncertainty. However, one thing was for certain: I refused to be another MS statistic.

The first step I took was to have my silver-mercury fillings removed and replaced with nontoxic plastic composite fillings. The mercury in the fillings was a factor in suppressing my immune system and partly responsible for the creation of MS.

The process of removal was no easy task for me. I could not tolerate any anesthesia or Novocain because they would produce an attack, which was like having a conscious epileptic seizure. I would spasm and tremor uncontrollably for several minutes and then become completely exhausted. Even though I wore a dental dam and a mask, I became severely ill after each extraction and replacement, as the mercury vapors and residue leached throughout my body. I flushed my system by drinking two quarts of red clover tea daily. This served to cleanse my blood, kidneys, and liver. I was barely able to lift my head up, and I experienced a couple of immune-response attacks daily throughout the two months that it took to complete the removal process. Mentally and physically I felt like a ninety-year-old witnessing the end of her life.

I endured the mercury removal, yet saw no signs of improvement. Instead, the progression of the MS attacks became more frequent and more severe. Afternoons into early evenings were my worst times because the body's level of cortisol, a hormone produced by the adrenal glands, typically drops during that period of time, and what little energy I had plummeted.

One night while lying on my mother's couch, with her and my stepfather close by, I felt my body shutting down and becoming completely paralyzed. My limbs were frozen, my breath slowed down, and I wasn't able to make a sound. Panic bubbled up in every cell of my body. I wanted to scream, but couldn't. As my lungs collapsed, I took my last breath and felt detached from my body. I felt warmth and light as I approached a tunnel of light. Time had stopped. I floated farther from my physical body and closer to the light. Then I heard a voice say, "Do you want to stay or go?"

I didn't want to go. Then there was silence. Seconds passed and I heard: "Stay! There is more for you to do."

Within a second of making the choice to stay, I shot back into my body, bolted off the couch, and let out a horrendous scream. My breathing had started again. My mother and stepfather leaped up and ran to my side. They had no idea what had just happened. They thought I was sleeping. My body was convulsing, my mind was like mush, and I couldn't formulate a word. Terror saturated every tissue as I returned from my "near-death" experience. As I wept in agony, I motioned for my mother to help me walk. I had to know I could still move. She assisted me around the living room while my body continued to spasm uncontrollably.

As terrified as I was to be back in my body, it was in that moment that I claimed my will to live and fight back with staunch courage and fierce tenacity. I vowed this illness would not destroy my life. The medical intuitive and Dr. Crook's work had exposed me to alternative treatments that had given me relief in the past—that is, when I stuck to them. I knew there was a way to overcome this insidious disease and I was determined to find it.

MY SEARCH FOR A CURE CONTINUES

Although I was physically limited, I could still read, so I began expanding my quest for a healing process. I read everything I could get my hands on with regard to the mind-body connection, nutrition, self-help, candidiasis, MS, and autoimmunity. The more I read, the more it became clear that suppressed childhood emotions and fear- and anger-based thoughts were factors in disease. It became crystal clear to me that treating the physical body alone was not enough to heal a chronic progressive disease.

My research took me back to the idea that yeast/fungal overgrowth was the major culprit in MS. Several follow-up sessions with my medical intuitive reinforced this. Through my research, I learned that candidiasis primarily targets the nerves and muscles, but can attack any tissue or organ, depending on the body's predisposition. The most common symptoms of candidiasis are indigestion, bloating, gas, fatigue, disorientation, poor memory, numbness, abdominal pain, constipation, attacks of anxiety, depression, irritability and shaking when hungry, lack of coordination, headaches, rashes, vaginal yeast infections, and urinary frequency.

In addition to Crook's *The Yeast Connection*, which made the correlation between yeast and autoimmune conditions, I found another book, *The Missing Diagnosis*, by C. Orian Truss, MD. Truss was a medical doctor who pioneered writing about candidiasis and presented case studies showing that yeast overgrowth negatively affects the body. In one such case study, he treated a female MS patient with Nystatin and diet modifications and she normalized to the extent that her neurologist found no more traces of MS.

So once again I started taking Nystatin, one 500,000-unit pill three times a day. I also adopted a very strict diet of no sugars, dairy, wheat, refined grains, red meat, and fermented or yeast-containing products. My goal was not only to eliminate candidiasis by removing the foods the yeast thrived on, but also to rebalance my digestion and absorption so my body could utilize the proper vitamins and minerals to do its job of rebuilding and regenerating.

The main supplements I took were vitamins C and E to support immunity and scavenge free radicals, and B-complex to help neurological function. I also took omega-3 fish oil and omega-6 evening primrose oil to repair my myelin sheath and drank a quart of red clover tea daily to cleanse my blood, liver, and kidneys. I may have also taken a couple of other supplements that I no longer remember. Since my knowledge in this area was limited, I instead focused on getting enough vitamins and minerals through variety in my diet.

CLEANING MY INTERNAL HOUSE

My most intense undertaking to help eradicate MS began when I decided to clean my internal house—emotionally, mentally, and spiritually. I started to challenge my outdated belief systems and embrace new ones, the main one being that I now believed my body could transform on a cellular level.

I began to peel away at my deep-seated fears. I realized how hard I was on myself and how my conditional love and self-judgment contributed to my ill health. I took responsibility for my illness and made getting well my most important priority.

My hardest realization was to accept that I had created this condition on a subconscious level. The subconscious mind is like a six-year-old. It has no discerning capability, loves repetition, and truly controls our daily actions and reactions. Mine was filled with a history of fear, anger, and low self-worth. Since

I had not addressed these subconscious patterns, I attracted new experiences with the same theme over and over again. As time passed, these experiences stressed and weakened my immune system. I knew I no longer wanted to be a victim, and accepting my accountability allowed me to tap into the power of knowing that I could make a different choice. I stepped into the driver's seat and started to believe I could create a new reality and release MS.

Despite my enthusiasm, I came up against much inner resistance. It was one thing to mentally grab onto new beliefs and thoughts, but it was another thing to feel them and to have my body agree. I discovered that physical matter, the body, didn't move as fast as my thoughts did. I wanted to incorporate other alternative therapies, such as acupuncture and massage, but my symptoms would worsen because of the hypersensitivity of my immune system.

Over time it became apparent that I was having difficulty breathing in Los Angeles because of the petroleum pollutants, so at age twenty-five I moved up to Sonoma County. This was a big step for me at such a vulnerable time in my life. I had made enough progress to walk and function on my own as long as I didn't push it. My threshold for stress had completely changed, and my body would let me know immediately by having an attack if I pushed it too far.

As soon as I moved, my body responded immediately to taking in more oxygen because of the improved air quality. I kept up with my regimen of eating healthy, drinking a lot of water and red clover tea, taking my supplements, and taking Nystatin. I started to take walks and noticed that I could go longer distances than before. But if I pushed it, my body would spasm and tremor.

Then there were days when my extreme nervous exhaustion made it impossible for me to get out of bed. The cloud of despair would overwhelm me again and I would cry and lie there wondering whether I would truly get well. But I learned to ride the tide of good days and bad days, and eventually I started to see more good days than bad.

A few months went by and I decided to challenge myself by accepting a part-time position at a bookstore. I did my best to take it day by day, but at times my fear of having attacks created more stress, which then brought about mild attacks. I kept pushing forward, and after six months of working and prevailing I decided to go back to college and enrolled at Sonoma State University. I changed my major from business marketing to psychology. I wanted to learn the deeper dimensions of who I was and how other people operated. During this period, attacks were triggered only by stress that was moderate to high. For example, I noticed more flare-ups during examination time.

By now, however, I knew the routine of caring for my body in a way that would get me through the down times. My fears were not so intense, but I still entertained thoughts like "Am I really getting better, or am I just fooling myself?" I would try to drown out these thoughts, as I wanted permanent remission. Knowing the disease could surface from time to time was not an option for me. I wanted a new body. I wanted cellular transformation, yet my body was not at the place I wanted it to be. I couldn't get past "believing" I could be healed to "knowing" that I would be.

One day I realized that health was a choice and that on an unconscious level I had chosen this disease as a way of discovering my own worth. That recognition took my breath away. The next natural realization was "I now have the power to choose a healthy body." This was a major breakthrough and a significant moment of enlightenment.

Although I was becoming clearer about my condition, I had some resistance and there was a tug of war going on inside of me. How could I have so much awareness and still feel powerless over killing my demons and changing my negative thinking?

PLUNGING THE DEPTHS

I was twenty-six when I flew back to Los Angeles for Thanksgiving. As we all began eating our Thanksgiving dinner, my grandmother on my father's side started choking. She turned purple and started gasping for air and waving her arms. I screamed for someone to help. My stepfather positioned himself behind her and administered the Heimlich maneuver until she coughed up a piece of turkey.

As she lay in an emergency room bed (her blood pressure had skyrocketed), I felt all my own terror about health start to gurgle in my throat. I could feel my stomach quivering with fear—hers and mine. I wanted to run out the door, but I remained by her side. The doctors said she was fine, so I took her back to my mother's house. But for the rest of the evening, while everyone was having fun, I couldn't shake the unsettling feelings, my grandmother's fears, and my fears. Little did I know how deeply my grandmother's choking episode would affect me.

November rolled into December. Finals were coming up and my stress level started to climb. I went out to lunch, ordered a couple of tacos, and had difficulty swallowing my first bite. Each bite was difficult to swallow. I thought maybe I was getting a sore throat. Dinnertime came and the same problem returned. Now I started to become worried and frustrated. I went to bed hoping this would all pass the next day, but my swallowing continued to be difficult. I forced the food down and was angry and perplexed at what was taking place. The difficulty continued meal after meal, but transformed into a fear of swallowing rather than a fear about the physical imbalance itself.

Oddly enough, this fear was in divine order, a step toward helping me get well. I didn't know it at the time, but it was the catalyst for releasing the suppressed, fear-based emotions I had been swallowing since childhood. Emotionally and mentally I was cleaning house, whether I liked it or not.

My energy dropped to zero. Between dealing with MS and now being afraid to swallow, I felt tightness and panic sitting on my chest all the time. I was in agony every waking hour and getting very little sleep. I was having a complete mental, physical, and spiritual breakdown. Unable to take care of myself, I moved back into my mother's house in Los Angeles.

Thoughts of suicide began to surface. The lack of sleep and food sent my mind into a tailspin of negative, uncontrollable thoughts. I ran over and over in my mind the events that had led up to all of this. I was angry with my grandmother for choking. I thought that if I hadn't developed the fear of swallowing, maybe I could deal with the MS. I fantasized about having a normal life, but my reality was anguish and despair. My state of mind and body was incredibly fragile. My body felt filled with electricity, ready to short-circuit at any moment. I was about to crack.

September 1, 1992, 4 a.m., at age twenty-seven, I tried to take my life.

On the way to the hospital I drifted in and out of consciousness, with my entire life flashing and flickering before me like a silent movie. I was admitted to the hospital right away as an attempted suicide. My left wrist needed stitches because the wounds were so deep. Tears coursed down my face. Never in my wildest dreams had I thought that this was how my life would turn out.

The doctor told my mother I would be put temporarily into a psychiatric detaining room until there was a space for me in the psychiatric ward. I was horrified. When they came to take me away I cried and begged for my mother to take me home. As they escorted me through a giant door, I turned and looked at her face, trying to capture every detail. The door closed and she was gone. I stood frozen in the abyss of the unknown.

I had entered the clinical world of drugs and psychiatric labels. Losing your mental faculties was a hundred times worse than losing your physical abilities. The doctors labeled me as being severely depressed.

As the days passed, I began to realize that the mind was the command station that ruled everything else in my physical and emotional existence. I could no longer ignore that thoughts created energy; that each thought—conscious or unconscious, spoken or unspoken—translated into electrical impulses that directed the control centers in my brain and central nervous system; and that the central nervous system controlled my every motion, cell, and feeling, and the actions I took every moment of every day. Simply put, my thoughts of suicide, fear, and negativity were manifesting in my reality.

RECOVERING

On day thirteen I was released from the hospital and sent to a halfway house. As I gathered my things, I heard another patient say to me, "Be good, or else you'll be back." I valued those words like gold because I loathed the thought of having to come back.

The head counselor at the halfway house was a middle-aged black woman who ran the show with an iron fist. She ended up being a crucial player in my life because she understood my anger and helped me get in touch with it as a means to save my life. We discovered that the root of the anger was my relationship with my mother and feeling abandoned by my father. The rage needed to come out, so day after day my counselors relentlessly stirred up the hornet's nest of emotions that lived inside me. Slowly, one by one, the layers began to peel away.

After two weeks I was transferred to another halfway house nearby. Getting through a day was tough, as I was deeply saddened and horrified by the sight of the other mentally ill patients. A few weeks into my stay, something miraculous took place as I routinely got ready for breakfast. Desperate, I decided to speak to God. I spoke the following words with conviction and passion from the depths of my soul: "God, I might be really screwed up right now, but I don't deserve this treatment anymore."

This realization and proclamation was life changing for me. It was in that very moment that I finally felt I was worth my existence. I now knew that worth was "inherent," based upon pure existence, and had nothing to do with how much money you make, what you do for a living, or if your family loves you. It was in that moment that I had an epiphany and reached out and seized my power. I decided right then I would no longer tolerate being a victim of low self-esteem and self-worth. I asked God to help me get better. I also asked for the strength to stand up for myself at any cost. And so my conversation with God turned into the foundation from which my hopes became a reality. I was released and sent home two weeks before Christmas.

SPIRALING UPWARD

Upon my release I started to see a psychotherapist. She was supportive and encouraging. With a big sigh of relief, I thought to myself, "I'm not crazy after all!" I understood that my break-down happened because in the process of transforming my body, I was going through a rebirth on every level. My therapist applauded me for my courage and reassured me that the worst was behind me.

By the end of February I was still struggling with my fear of swallowing. One afternoon I was mindlessly flipping through the cable channels and I stopped on the public access station. A Russian hypnotherapist was being interviewed. As I watched, it was as if someone grabbed me around the neck and said, "Go see this man!"

I made an appointment immediately. Peter was confident and told me that before long my fear of swallowing and other negative patterns would be gone. For the first time in months, I let down my guard and relaxed. I went deep into a hypnotic state and didn't even remember what was said during the session. When we were done, I had an absolute knowingness that I was going to get better. I had finally gone beyond believing. I "knew" I was being healed.

Within a month, it was as if a miracle had happened. I was stronger, healthier, and more centered than I had ever been in my life. My thoughts were focused and positive. I was able to recognize old behaviors and feel neutral rather than negative emotionally. It was as if someone had cleared the cobwebs and removed my self-sabotaging ways.

I was healthy inside and out, able to swallow and to live each day without nagging fear. Because my psychological body was now much more whole and I had taken all the physical steps up to that point—Nystatin, supplements, and the detoxi-fication of my body—the transformation was solidified and my MS was reversed.

Soon afterwards I was able to stop taking Nystatin and

replaced it with Candida Cleanse to maintain balance. I continued to eat healthy, take supplements, drink red clover tea, and exercise regularly.

As I felt better spiritually and emotionally, I witnessed how my physical body remained healthy for longer periods of time. I had not experienced an attack in months. I started to feel better overall, without numbness and tingling in parts of my body. I became active and started to play social sports. I felt normal.

Feeling capable of working, I went back to the record company I had previously worked for. My expansion as a person became more evident, and after a while I grew restless and left the job within a year. I sensed that there was much more to my healing journey than just getting better, and that within the experience was a calling to take the next step.

I moved to Taos, New Mexico, and became inspired by the idea of writing about the incredible journey I had been on and how I had healed myself. Writing was challenging, and my mind started to grab onto a larger prospect of becoming a healer. So I went back to school to become a naturopath and clinical hypnotherapist.

I graduated from the International Society of Naturopathy as a naturopathic doctor and became a certified clinical hypnotherapist from the Holmes Hypnotherapy School. At thirty-three I opened my own practice in Los Angeles. A couple of years later I added to my credentials by becoming a certified iridologist from Bernard Jensen's International Iridology Practitioners Association, and by becoming a certified nutritional consultant from the American Association of Nutritional Consultants.

Initially, as a practitioner, I woke up almost every day and watched to see if my neurological symptoms were gone. To my pleasure, they were, and continue to be. I have not experienced the slightest sign or symptom of MS in the last twenty years.

TRIUMPH

I do not underestimate the journey I have walked. I have undergone a complete metamorphosis. For the longest time I could not see the light, but I remained diligent in my efforts to reach my destination. I now know that in the worst of times I was guided and protected. I know the power of God.

My complete transformation could not have occurred without having challenged and addressed each component of my existence. Just following the diet, taking an antifungal and supplements, and having my mercury fillings removed would not have been enough. It was also necessary for me to examine and release my fear-based childhood experiences. To take these steps required awareness, self-acceptance, and taking responsibility for my physically ravaged body.

My relationships with those around me have changed, specifically with my parents. I now understand that the dynamics in which I grew up ignited my strength and courage and made me who I am today. I can now interact with them from a place of confidence and neutrality. They were my best teachers and I know they did the best they could. I understand that because their childhoods were difficult, certain negative patterns and cycles carried on. Humbly, and in hindsight, I also know each of us would have made different choices where mistakes were made if we were able to at the time.

I owe the Western medical community a debt of gratitude for having pushed me to the limits to go beyond their protocols and find answers. Turning myself into a guinea pig had its pluses, for I learned firsthand that the body can rejuvenate and repair itself, even in the face of great adversity.

The attacking agent for MS—or any disease—is not simply yeast, or a virus, or an organ system that has failed. It is much more than that. The cause is a culmination of the history of each individual's thoughts, emotions, stress levels, spiritual connection, genetics, diet, and environmental factors. The body's cellular memory stores every element, and part of regaining health and restoring vitality means uncovering each one and releasing it. The body inherently seeks health and balance. It is only when the toxins we are harboring overpower our body's ability to remove them that autoimmune disease occurs.

In Dr. Andrew Weil's book *Spontaneous Healing*, he states: "One of the most effective ways to neutralize medical pessimism is to find someone who had the same problem you do and is now healed. Whenever I come across people who have solved serious health problems, I ask them if they will allow me from time to time to send similarly affected patients for advice and guidance."[2]

For the last fifteen years I have helped thousands of clients reclaim their health. In Part Three you will read the success stories of some of my clients. My expertise is in my ability to help others find the root causes of their disease. My mission is to impart to those who are struggling with this illness, as I was, that remission and reversal are possible. With determination, patience, the proper protocol, and the "knowing," it is within your power to transform the body and the mind.

THE REAL CAUSE OF MULTIPLE SCLEROSIS

MS AND THE CANDIDA CONNECTION

WHAT IS MULTIPLE SCLEROSIS?

Multiple sclerosis is an autoimmune disease of the central nervous system (CNS), which includes the brain and spinal cord. It affects more than three million people worldwide, at least half a million of them in the United States. Women are twice as likely to develop MS as men. The disease occurs more often in temperate climates, such as the United States and Northern Europe, and usually strikes adults in their twenties to forties.

A variety of tests are used to diagnose MS, including magnetic resonance imaging (MRI); electroencephalography (EEG); spinal taps; blood assay tests; and visual-, somato-sensory-, and brain-stem-evoked potentials (EPs—measure the electrical signals that result from sensory stimuli).

MS is an inflammatory condition that destroys myelin (the white fatty tissue that insulates the nerves) and slows or stops the conduction of nerve impulses. The myelin becomes inflamed and detached from the nerve fibers and eventually turns into hardened patches of scar tissue (scleroses) that form over the fibers. These lesions can appear in various areas of the brain and spinal cord. This demyelination can also cause what is called "cross-talk" between the nerve fibers, which disrupts normal nerve signals and produces many of the symptoms of MS.

SYMPTOMS AND CLASSIFICATIONS

There is not one set standard or classic case that defines MS. Symptoms include fatigue, spasticity, paralysis, blurred and double vision, numbness, lack of coordination, tingling, dizziness, speech and swallowing impairments, bladder and bowel problems, sensitivity to heat, cognitive dysfunction (memory loss, changes in thinking or perception, and loss of focus and problem-solving ability), sexual dysfunction, pain, and tremors.

Multiple sclerosis is classified into five categories:

- Benign: usually one or two attacks with complete recovery. This form does not worsen.
- Relapsing-remitting: unpredictable relapses (attacks, exacerbations) during which new symptoms appear or existing ones worsen. Flare-ups are followed by periods of remission.
- Primary-progressive: from the first appearance of symptoms, neurological function deteriorates, without periods of remission.
- Secondary-progressive: begins as relapsing-remitting MS and is followed by a stage of continuous deterioration later in the course of the disease.
- Progressive-relapsing: primary progressive MS with the addition of sudden episodes of new symptoms or a worsening of existing ones.

THE WESTERN MEDICAL PROTOCOL

Western medicine states that MS is incurable. Millions of dollars have been spent in research, most of which points to an infection, or perhaps a virus, as the cause, but nothing concrete has been identified.

Pharmaceutical companies have developed drugs designed to reduce the symptoms and slow or stop the progression of MS:

- Intravenous corticosteroids such as prednisone and Solu-Medrol are prescribed to reduce inflammation and shorten the duration of flare-ups.
- Baclofen, Zanaflex, Klonopin, and Lioresal are administered to treat spasticity and pain.
- Amantadine and Provigil are used for fatigue management.
- Antivert is used for vertigo.
- Ampyra is used to help with walking.
- Ditropan and Tegretol are both prescribed for urinary problems.
- Botox is prescribed for urinary incontinence.
- Prozac, Zoloft, Celexa, and Effexor are used to minimize depression and anxiety.
- Beta interferons such as Avonex, Betaseron, and Rebif are genetically engineered copies of proteins used to help the body fight viral infection and improve the regulation of the immune system. (In July 2012, the *Journal of the American Medical Association* published a research study stating that treatment with disease-modifying beta interferon drugs such as Avonex, Betaseron, Extavia, and Rebif did not slow down the progression of MS.)

- Copaxone, a synthetic drug made up of four amino acids, is designed to mimic the reactive portion of myelin that the immune system destroys.
- Naltrexone is used to boost the immune system by briefly blocking opioid receptors, which increases endorphin and enkephalin production.
- Even chemotherapy drugs such as Novantrone, Cytoxan, Alemtuzumab, Rituximab, Daclizumab, and Imuran are used to treat MS.
- Tysabri, formerly known as Antegren, was voluntarily suspended by the makers in 2005 due to a couple of fatalities, but is back on the market and has caused twenty more deaths since 2007.
- Oral medications to treat relapsing-remitting MS (RRMS) have surfaced, making compliance easier for the patient. Gilenya is a new class of medication called a sphingosine 1-phosphate receptor modulator, which is thought to act by retaining certain white blood cells (lymphocytes) in the lymph nodes, thereby preventing those cells from crossing the blood-brain barrier into the central nervous system.
- Laquinimod (oral) is a quinolone compound that affects immune response pathways of white blood cells Th1 (Type 1 helper T cells) and Th2 (Type 2 helper T cells).
- Aubagio (teriflunomide, oral) mimics DNA and blocks and interferes with normal DNA synthesis needed for rapidly dividing autoimmune cells.
- Tecfidera (fumaric acid salts, oral), formerly called BG-12, has been used for psoriasis in the UK for several years and sounds more promising as a treatment for MS than any of the drugs listed above. It is the first compound to activate the Nrf2 pathway, which

defends against oxidative-stress-induced neuronal death, protects the blood-brain barrier, and supports maintenance of myelin integrity in the central nervous system. Unlike most MS drugs, Tecfidera is not just based on suppression or the modulation of the immune system; it detoxifies damaging free radicals released during the inflammation processes and thus supports the survival of nerve cells.

- Intravenous immunoglobulin (IVIG) is made from antibodies that have been filtered from the pooled blood of over a thousand donors. Immunoglobulins are proteins that function as antibodies and are secreted by white blood cells and plasma cells. IVIG has shown temporary improvement in neurological diseases by increasing the action of some parts of the immune system and decreasing the action of others.

- Plasma exchange (plasmapheresis) involves drawing some of a patient's blood, removing the plasma (the liquid portion), and replacing it with another solution, typically albumin or a synthetic fluid with properties like plasma. The blood is then returned to the patient's body. This procedure removes circulating antibodies, which are thought to be active in autoimmune disease. It may temporarily restore neurological function in people with sudden severe attacks of MS-related disability who don't respond to high doses of steroid treatment. However, it has not been shown to be effective for secondary-progressive MS or primary-progressive MS.

All of these drugs have side effects. Mild reactions include flu-like symptoms, nausea, headaches, and muscle aches. More severe side effects are liver damage, convulsions, blood clots, suicide, hallucinations, and paralysis. The main MS drugs used to slow down the progression of MS—beta interferons, Tysabri, and Copaxone—have only a 30 percent efficacy. However, Tecfidera has been shown to have a higher efficacy of about 44 percent when taken twice daily, and 51 percent when taken three times a day. It also has fewer and milder side effects than the other drugs.

The annual cost to the consumer for the MS drugs currently on the market is between $10,000 and $14,000 ($40,000 to $60,000 a year if you are uninsured). Unfortunately, pharmaceutical companies apparently have a more important mission than finding a cure. Their main priority is to make sure that their revenues continue to soar.

I am not anti-Western medicine, yet there is so much more we can do using safe means to address the underlying causes of the disease, which are inflammation and infection in the body. What's important for you to know is that there are many ways to get to the light at the end of the tunnel. Some people do better integrating pharmaceuticals with alternative therapies, and some improve by just implementing alternative lifestyle changes. There is no right or wrong way to heal, and you can always change your mind during the course of your healing.

One suggestion to help you decide whether to use medication is to ask yourself this question, "Will I have more fear about what is going to happen to my body if I don't take a drug?" If the answer is yes, it is probably best to take the medication because the stress caused by your fear will contribute to the crumbling of your health. If you are more afraid to be on medication, you have answered your own question. The key is to educate yourself so that you can make empowered choices and to remember that you are in the driver's seat. The bottom line, why settle for alleviating symptoms when you can get to the root cause?

RESEARCH

A procedure called Liberation Treatment, which uses balloon venoplasty on veins (much like an angioplasty that is done on arteries), was being used in the U.S. for two years by some doctors to treat MS patients. However, in May 2012 the FDA prohibited its practice except in approved clinical studies to evaluate its safety and effectiveness.

The treatment was fashioned after the research of Dr. Paolo Zamboni of Italy, who published the results of his study of sixty-five MS patients in June 2009. He discovered they had chronic cerebrospinal venous insufficiency (CCSVI), an abnormality in blood drainage from the brain and spinal cord that may contribute to nervous system damage in MS. He found the veins that transport blood from the brain were twisted and blocked. This causes blood to flow backwards into the brain, depositing high levels of iron. Deposits of iron can be toxic to the brain and may set off a series of immune reactions leading to MS.

Stem cell research involving transplants of embryonic and adult stem cells is also still underway. Stem cells are injected into the bloodstream with the hope of repairing nerve damage to the brain and myelin sheath. Bone marrow stem-cell transplantation, which replaces the body's faulty immune memory with "cleansed" immune cells, is another approach being researched.

An experimental therapy using Tovaxin (T cell vaccination) was granted fast-track designation by the FDA in 2011, and is in clinical trials as a first-line treatment for secondary-progressive MS. The treatment uses the patient's blood to create a vaccine using his or her own immune cells. The cells are irradiated to render them unable to divide, but capable of evoking an immune response, and are then injected into the patient.

All of the above treatments may have some value, but they do not address the underlying cause of the disease.

THE HIDDEN CAUSE OF MS

Candida albicans overgrowth and its by-products (mycotoxins) are the primary cause of MS. However, this pathogenic (disease-producing) yeast/fungus is continually ignored by Western medicine, even though it is the missing key to reversing MS.

Candida albicans is a harmless yeast that naturally lives in everyone's body: men, women, and children alike. In a healthy body, it lives symbiotically in a balanced environment in the gastrointestinal tract, on the mucous membranes, and on the skin. Unfortunately, this harmless yeast can overgrow and turn into an opportunistic pathogen.

As Dr. Michael Goldberg states: "Because it is a commensal organism [one that benefits from another organism without damaging or benefiting it] present in virtually all human beings from birth, it is ideally positioned to take immediate advantage of any weakness or debility in the host, and probably has few equals in the variety and severity of the infections for which it is responsible."[1]

Candida overgrowth and its mycotoxins can attack any organ or system in your body. The attack is relentless, twenty-four hours a day, until treated. If not arrested, the yeast, a single-celled organism, will change form into a pathogenic fungus with roots and cause myriad symptoms. (Throughout the book, I will be using the words *yeast* and *fungus* interchangeably.)

This fungus burrows its roots into the intestinal lining and creates leaky gut—porous openings in the gut lining—which allows the yeast/fungus and its by-products to escape into the bloodstream. This systemic yeast/fungal infection is called *candidiasis*. According to an article in the journal *Science*, "*Candida albicans* is the most common human systemic pathogen, causing both mucosal and systemic infections, particularly in immunocompromised people."[2]

LIFESTYLE FACTORS THAT CAUSE YEAST OVERGROWTH

The major causes of *Candida albicans* overgrowth are antibiotics, steroids (e.g., cortisone and prednisone), birth control pills, estrogen replacement therapy, poor diet, chemotherapy, radiation, heavy metals, alcohol overuse, recreational drugs, and stress. Other contributing factors include heavy metals in our silver amalgam fillings and the lead and cadmium in polluted air. All of the above directly or indirectly destroy the good bacteria in our gastrointestinal tract (GI tract), allowing yeast to take over.

Yeast overgrowth thrives in the presence of diets high in refined sugars, refined carbohydrates, dairy products, alcohol, and processed foods, and as the result of high stress levels. Acute and chronic stress elevate cortisol, a hormone produced and secreted by the adrenal glands. Excessive cortisol, in turn, raises blood sugar. The fungus doesn't care whether the increased sugar in your body is due to eating a candy bar or to having an episode of extreme stress; it will use the sugar as fuel to reproduce itself.

Once an imbalance occurs, yeast continue to multiply as they are fed by sugar in any form—alcohol, desserts, white flour, dairy products like milk and cheese, and elevated sugar levels caused by high stress. As years go by, mild to severe health conditions appear. It is easy to see why the incidence of candidiasis is so high—the main contributing factors are various mainstream Western medicine protocols, rampant poor diet, and the stress overload so prevalent in our society today.

Western medicine may deny that yeast cause these myriad conditions, but the truth is that fungal toxins—the by-products produced by the yeast—disrupt cellular communication. Once that happens, inflammation and infection settle wherever we are genetically weak.

THE DRAWBACKS OF TAKING ANTIBIOTICS

It takes only one dose of antibiotics in your lifetime to raise your yeast levels and create imbalances in your body. If you last took a course of antibiotics when you were ten years old, a poor diet and high stress levels will continue to feed the yeast over time until you begin to feel symptomatic. Think about how many times you've taken antibiotics—not to mention the antibiotics you ingest from consuming dairy and animal products.

North America (especially the United States and Canada) and pockets of Europe have the highest numbers of people with candidiasis because Western medicine's standard protocol is to use antibiotic therapy for common infections.

A vicious cycle starts with the use of antibiotics (see Figure 2.1). For example, you have a cold or the flu and you visit your doctor, who prescribes antibiotics. The problem starts right there because colds and flu are viral infections, not bacterial infections, which are what antibiotics are designed to treat. Antibiotics are useless against colds and flu, yet many doctors prescribe them anyway. When you take the antibiotic it kills both the good and bad bacteria in your gastrointestinal tract because it cannot distinguish between them. Antibiotics do not affect *Candida albicans*, so without friendly bacteria like *Lactobacillus acidophilus* and *Bifidobacteria* to keep the *Candida albicans* under control, the candida will now multiply.

There is no question that antibiotics have saved thousands of lives, but we've pushed a good thing too far by overprescribing these medications. Overuse also creates "super germs" that

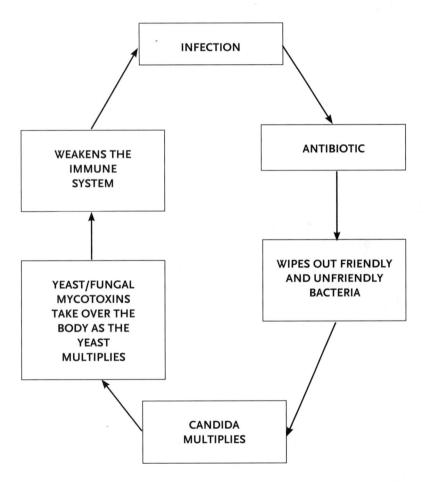

Source: Reprinted courtesy of William G. Crook, MD, *The Yeast Connection Handbook* (Jackson, TN: Professional Books, 2000). Used with permission.

FIGURE 2.1. The Vicious Cycle of Antibiotic Overuse

are resistant to common antibiotics, so germs that could once be killed off have now become life threatening.

CANDIDA'S TOXIC BY-PRODUCTS

Once candida is in an overgrowth state, the body has to deal not only with the overgrowth but also with the toxic by-products, or mycotoxins, that *Candida albicans* puts out—"79 at latest count,"[3] according to C. Orian Truss, MD. All of these weaken your immune system and attack the myelin sheath in those with MS.

Mycotoxins are neurotoxins that destroy and decompose tissues and organs. They are so powerful that they upset the very communication of cell interactions, disrupt RNA and DNA synthesis, damage and destroy neurons, are carcinogenic, and cause ataxia (lack of coordination) and even convulsions. These pernicious yeast toxins confuse body systems, which accounts for the cross-wiring problems of your immune system once you have MS.

Candida toxins commonly get through the gut lining when it becomes leaky and then enter the bloodstream. In a healthy system, the liver detoxifies the blood. However, if the liver's detoxification ability is impaired due to inadequate nutrition and toxic overload, these toxins will settle in other organs and tissues, such as the brain, nervous system, joints, skin, and so forth. Over time, chronic disease will occur.

One of the major toxins produced from *Candida albicans* is acetaldehyde (a by-product of alcohol metabolism), which the liver converts into a harmless substance. However, if there is an excess of acetaldehyde and the liver becomes oversaturated, it is released into the bloodstream, creating feelings of intoxication, brain fog, vertigo, and loss of equilibrium. Acetaldehyde alters the structure of red blood cells and compromises the transportation pathways whereby materials are delivered to feed the dendrites (nerve cell extensions), which causes the dendrites to atrophy and die off.

In addition, acetaldehyde creates a deficiency of thiamine (vitamin B1), a vitamin that is critical for brain and nerve function and essential for the production of acetylcholine, one of the brain's major neurotransmitters (see Table 2.1). This deficiency brings on emotional apathy, depression, fatigue, insomnia, confusion, and memory loss.

Acetaldehyde also depletes niacin (vitamin B3), which is key to helping the cells burn fat and sugar for energy. Niacin plays an important role in the production of serotonin (a

TABLE 2.1. Damage from Acetaldehyde

Acetaldehyde Damages Brain Function

- Impaired memory
- Decreased ability to concentrate ("brain fog")
- Depression
- Slowed reflexes
- Lethargy and apathy
- Heightened irritability
- Decreased mental energy
- Increased anxiety and panic
- Decreased sensory acuity
- Increased tendency to alcohol and sugar
- Decreased sex drive
- Increased PMS and breast swelling/tenderness in women

Source: James A. South, MA, *Vitamin Research Products Nutritional News*, July 1997.

neurotransmitter that affects mood and sleep) and in the production of a coenzyme that breaks down alcohol. Acetaldehyde
also reduces enzymes in the body that help to produce energy
in all cells, including brain cells.

Gliotoxin, another mycotoxin, deactivates important enzymes that move toxins through the body and also causes DNA
changes in the white blood cells that suppress the immune system. As your immune system continues to weaken from yeast/
fungus and mycotoxins, more infections arise and you end up
at the doctor's office again—being prescribed more antibiotics
and perpetuating the vicious cycle.

CANDIDA'S PREFERRED TARGETS

Candida albicans primarily targets the nerves and muscles, yet
it can attack any tissue or organ, depending on your body's genetic predisposition (see Table 2.2). Women are more affected
than men because of their anatomy and hormone fluctuations,
but men are vulnerable as well. Note that candidiasis can be
transmitted back and forth between sexual partners.

To understand how candida penetrates through your system, think of your body as having two skins of protection that
keep out foreign invaders. One is the outside skin and the other
is your inside skin, which starts in your nasal passages and
runs all the way down to your rectum. This tissue is the same
from top to bottom, and if it becomes inflamed or irritated, the
membranes become more porous, allowing foreign invaders
to enter the bloodstream and to break through the blood-brain
barrier.

World-renowned neurologist David Perlmutter says this
about candida's connection to MS:

The frequency of focal white matter lesions in patients with inflammatory bowel disease is almost as high as that in patients with multiple sclerosis. These findings provide convincing evidence supporting that relationship between gut abnormalities and brain pathology. New research clearly reveals a very important relationship between MS and problems in the digestive system like inflammatory bowel disease, yeast overgrowth, and low levels of healthful bacteria. This organism (*Candida albicans*) has been associated with hyper-immune diseases and specifically MS.[4]

Candida albicans and its mycotoxins accumulate in the central nervous system, where they attack and create lesions on the myelin sheath. At this point the whole body is saturated with toxins, which causes the secondary systems of other parts of the body to deteriorate. As the immune system continues to weaken from the constant attack of fungus, its by-products, and inflammatory agents, the body is thrown into a catabolic state and the tissues, muscles, and organs break down. Chronic toxicity overtaxes the immune system, which then loses its ability to function and starts attacking itself. This is a simplified explanation of how autoimmune disease is created.

Dr. Perlmutter routinely screens for yeast overgrowth and integrates anti-yeast treatment when working with his multiple sclerosis patients. He states:

The possible link between various autoimmune diseases and infection with the yeast *Candida albicans* has been described by well-respected researchers over the past two decades. We believe that these data provide compelling evidence that candidiasis may, at the very

TABLE 2.2 Yeast/Fungal Overgrowth
(conditions caused directly or indirectly by overgrowth)

Autoimmune Diseases
ALS (Lou Gehrig's Disease)
Chronic Fatigue Syndrome
Fibromyalgia
HIV/AIDS
Hodgkin's Disease
Leukemia
Lupus
Multiple Sclerosis
Muscular Dystrophy
Myasthenia Gravis
Rheumatoid Arthritis
Sarcoidosis
Scleroderma

Blood System
Chronic Infections
Iron Deficiency
Thrombocytopenic Purpura

Cancer

Cardiovascular System
Endocarditis
Pericarditis
Mitral Valve Prolapse
Valve Problems

Digestive System
Anorexia Nervosa
Bloating/Gas
Carbohydrate/Sugar Cravings
Colitis
Constipation/Diarrhea
Crohn's Disease
Dysbiosis
Food Allergies
Gastritis
Heartburn
Intestinal Pain
Irritable Bowel Syndrome
Leaky Gut
Malabsorption/Maldigestion

**Respiratory System/
Ears/Eyes/Mouth**
Asthma
Bronchitis
Dizziness
Earaches
Environmental Allergies/
Chemical Sensitivities
Hay Fever
Oral Thrush
Sinusitis

Endocrine System
Adrenal/Thyroid Failure
Diabetes
Hormonal Imbalances
Hypoglycemia
Insomnia
Over-/Underweight

Skin
Acne
Diaper Rash
Dry Skin and Itching
Eczema
Hives
Hair Loss
Leprosy
Liver Spots
Psoriasis

Nervous System
Alcoholism
Anxiety
Attention Deficit Disorder
Autism
Brain Fog
Depression
Headaches
Hyperactivity
Hyperirritability
Learning Difficulties
Manic-Depressive Disorder
Memory Loss
Migraines
Schizophrenia
Suicidal Tendencies

Urinary/Reproductive Systems
Cystitis
Endometriosis
Fibroids
Impotence
Loss of Libido
Menstrual Irregularities
PMS
Prostatitis
Sexually Transmitted Diseases
Urethritis
Yeast Vaginal Infections

Virus
Epstein-Barr Virus

least, be a frequent occurrence in patients with multiple sclerosis. In addition, these data seem to indicate that intestinal dysbiosis [an imbalance of the good and bad bacteria in the gut] may be common in MS patients. We now routinely perform serum analysis for candida immune complexes and candida antibodies (IgG, IgM, and IgA) as well as a comprehensive digestive stool analysis on our MS patients. Our success in reducing fatigue in MS with treatments designed specifically to reduce candida activity lends further support for the suggested relationship between MS-related fatigue and candida activity. Further we suggest that intestinal dysbiosis may play a pivotal role with respect to the actual pathogenesis of MS as an autoimmune disease entity.[5]

Another neurologist, R. Scott Heath, did a study with MS patients by putting them on an anti-candida diet and Diflucan. Heath said that "no patients experienced exacerbations while on diet and Diflucan."[6]

EMOTIONAL AND MENTAL IMBALANCES

Emotional and mental imbalances are common occurrences with *Candida albicans* overgrowth. Depression and anxiety are almost constant components of systemic illness related to chronic yeast growth in the tissues. The reason, as described by J. P. Nolan in an article in the journal *Hepatology*, is the link between the gut and the brain: "An individual's ability to protect against brain-active substances depends upon the status of his or her intestinal flora, GI mucosal function and hepatic (liver) detoxification ability."[7] This means that when leaky gut is present and the liver is overstressed, the door is open for toxins to reach the brain via the bloodstream.

Unfortunately, too many physicians assume that all mental or emotional imbalances have psychological causes, such as neuroses or psychoses, rather than brain-related causes, as Truss points out in *The Missing Diagnosis*:

> I would like to make a special plea that we speak of manifestations of abnormal brain function not as "mental symptoms" but as "brain symptoms." Inherent in the term "mental symptom" is the connotation that somehow "the mind" is a separate entity from the brain, that "mental" symptoms are occurring (at least initially) in a brain that is functioning normally chemically and physiologically. We speak of kidney, liver, or intestinal symptoms when abnormal function manifests itself in these organs, but we use the term "mental symptoms" rather than "brain symptoms" when a similar problem occurs with brain physiology.[8]

If you have MS, anxiety and/or depression can be debilitating. Know that these symptoms are due to a chemical imbalance caused by an overtaxed immune system combined with the psychological stress of having a serious condition. Your mental and emotional imbalances are therefore to be treated, not ignored or discounted.

WESTERN MEDICINE'S DENIAL

To this day, Western medicine does not recognize intestinal and systemic candidiasis as a health condition. Don't be surprised if you take this information to your neurologist and he or she dismisses it or tells you that you are crazy. It's odd that doctors who routinely recognize and treat *Candida albicans* overgrowth in cases of oral thrush, vaginal infections, and HIV/AIDS in patients whose immune systems are severely compromised refuse to see MS in the same light, since it is also a condition of a compromised immune system.

With antibiotics, hormone replacement drugs, birth control pills, and steroid drugs accounting for millions of dollars in prescriptions written each year, doctors are going to be the last ones to acknowledge that the drugs they so freely prescribe are actually creating the problem, or that intestinal candidiasis even exists. There are some good doctors who will treat intestinal and systemic candidiasis, but they are few and far between.

MAKING THE CONNECTION: CANDIDA AND MS

All or most autoimmune diseases are caused by yeast/fungal toxins. One difference between the illnesses has to do with whether the fungal toxins are the primary or secondary cause. For people with MS, they are the primary attacking agent. The similarities between candidiasis and MS are these:

- MS affects more women than it does men; so does candidiasis.
- MS symptoms are due to the impairment of the nervous system (causing numbness, tingling, fatigue, poor coordination, urinary frequency, depression, and erratic vision). These are also the symptoms of chronic candidiasis.
- The most common symptom in both conditions is fatigue.
- Intestinal dysbiosis (an imbalance between the good

and bad bacteria in the gut) and leaky gut are common to both.

- Both conditions suppress the immune system and cause the body to be in an inflammatory state.
- Candidiasis patients have vitamin and mineral deficiencies, as do people with MS.
- Food allergies and gluten intolerance are common in both conditions.
- Both conditions have been linked with the Epstein-Barr virus.
- Finally, both conditions will respond positively to dietary changes and an antifungal regime.

You can eliminate MS by changing your lifestyle and your diet, eliminating heavy metals from the body, reducing stress, and changing geographical location if necessary. Addressing these factors has been shown to account for periods of lapses and remission of symptoms. No matter what your stage of MS, treatment of candidiasis is essential to turning your condition around.

The correlation between candidiasis and MS does not currently have a lot of scientific research to back it up simply because it hasn't been done. However, the connection is not to be overlooked. It is the missing piece of the puzzle you have been looking for—*Candida albicans* overgrowth is the invisible catalyst that causes this "incurable" disease.

CHAPTER THREE

SECONDARY FACTORS THAT CONTRIBUTE TO MS

FACTORS THAT BRING ABOUT DISEASE

In today's world, there are more factors than ever before that are affecting your body in ways that bring about disease: the depleted foods you eat, the synthetic chemicals and toxins you absorb, and the overload of emotional and mental stress you endure.

When your capacity to eliminate toxicity becomes overburdened, disease sets in. Your doctor gives you drugs, but these only add more toxins to the body and cover up symptoms without getting to the root cause. Yes, there are times when drugs are useful, but most are designed to only alleviate symptoms.

The point is to move beyond symptoms and to ignite your body's own defense mechanisms so it can heal itself. When toxins and distress are eliminated, and vitamins and minerals are balanced, the body can do its job of repairing itself. Preventing disease is not only about eliminating outside factors such as germs that you pick up. Rather it's about tending to your internal environment so that it does not become compromised and produce favorable conditions for microbes such as bacteria, viruses, parasites, and yeast to take over. Even Louis Pasteur, the famous French scientist who discovered the germ theory, said near the end of his life that it was more important to look to the body's internal environment than to germs as the cause of disease.

While candidiasis is the underlying and primary cause of MS, there are secondary contributors that are worth examining. These include amalgam fillings, viruses, vaccinations, poor diet, food allergies, physical trauma, psychological stress, and environmental toxicity.

Silver-Mercury (Amalgam) Fillings

Silver-mercury fillings consist of 52 percent mercury. The remaining metals are silver, tin, copper, and traces of zinc. Numerous studies have shown that amalgam fillings suppress the immune system and can create illness (see Table 3.1). MS is one of the primary conditions linked to mercury poisoning.

Many countries in Europe ban the use of amalgam fillings, but the American Dental Association still stands firm in proclaiming that they are safe. Mercury is a poisonous metal that accumulates in the nerves, brain, kidneys, and livers of those exposed to it. Most of us received amalgam fillings at a young age and still have them in our mouths as adults. Amalgams came into use primarily because of their durability. The problem is that over time there is wear and tear on these fillings, which causes leaching. An article in the *Townsend Letter* states: "The mercury escapes from fillings in the form of vapor created by chewing. It then enters the bloodstream and is delivered to all parts of the body, including the brain. It is our conclusion that mercury toxicity is an autoimmune disorder. Mercury is the most toxic nonradioactive element on earth, and an amalgam filling contains 52 percent mercury."[1]

TABLE 3.1 Symptoms of Chronic, Low-Dose Mercury Exposure

- Abdominal pain
- Abnormal reflexes
- Adverse outcome of pregnancy
- Anorexia (lack of appetite)
- Anuria (cessation of urine production)
- Ataxia (difficulty in moving)
- Disturbed gait
- Erethism (nervousness, irritability, mood instability, blushing)
- Excessive salivation
- Gastroenteritis (stomach upset)
- Gingivitis (inflammation of the gums)
- Glioblastoma (brain cancer)
- Immune system dysfunction
- Impaired hearing
- Impaired nerve conduction
- Infertility
- Mouth pain
- Nephritis (kidney disease leading to kidney failure)
- Personality change
- Pneumonitis (lung disease)
- Paresthesia (prickling, tingling, or creeping sensations on the skin)
- Renal damage
- Speech disorders
- Suicidal tendency
- Tremor
- Uremia (appearance of urine products in the blood)
- Visual disturbances
- Vomiting

Not everyone with MS has amalgam fillings, so this is only one part of the puzzle. I would recommend that those with MS who have amalgam fillings get them removed. This is a factor that you will need to examine in consult with your health practitioner and your dentist. I discuss this in greater detail in Chapter 9.

Viruses And Bacteria

Almost all of us have been exposed to viruses as children, though not everyone gets sick from them. The strength of your immune system determines whether viruses take hold during your lifetime.

When yeast overgrowth is present and the fungus and its by-products move through your system, your body is depleted of oxygen. This imbalanced ecology creates a perfect breeding ground for bacterial, viral, and parasitical infections.

Several viruses and bacteria show up more consistently than others in the blood work of those with MS. They are *borrelia burgdorferi*, which is the agent responsible for Lyme disease and is transmitted through tick bites; human herpes virus 6 (HHV-6), which commonly causes roseola in infants; chlamydia pneumonia, commonly involved in respiratory infections; cytomegalovirus (CMV); and Epstein-Barr virus, which can bring on mononucleosis.

In an article entitled "Viruses and Multiple Sclerosis" in the December 2001 issue of the *Journal of the American Medical Association*, Donald H. Gilden, MD, cited findings that the Epstein-Barr virus may also increase the risk of MS.[2] This virus often surfaces in those with candida overgrowth, as the yeast toxins produce a suitable environment for the virus to take over. Thus, candida overgrowth is the precursor to the Epstein-Barr virus becoming active.

When you have MS, these infections need to be considered as potentially present and dealt with. By treating candidiasis, you will also treat viruses, bacteria, and parasites.

Vaccinations

Vaccinations are controversial, to say the least. The purpose of a vaccination is to create resistance to a disease by injecting a weakened or killed microorganism of the same disease. Unfortunately, vaccinations can cause or contribute to several severe complications, including autism, allergies, sudden infant death syndrome, and autoimmune disease.

The risk is heightened because thimerosal, a water-soluble, cream-colored crystalline powder that is 49.6 percent mercury by weight, is used as a preservative in many vaccines. As I discussed above, mercury is highly toxic. Other additives in vaccines are aluminum, formaldehyde, and monosodium glutamate (MSG), all of which are neurotoxins.

Vaccination complications are not a new phenomenon. In the early and mid-1950s penicillin came into common use as an antibiotic, and at the same time the first polio vaccinations were being administered. The indiscriminate use of the two set the stage for them to interact and cause fungal infections. The repercussions were retroviruses that surfaced later in adulthood. Post-vaccination damage is not always immediately obvious. It can take weeks, months, and even years to show up in the body. In 1967, the *British Medical Journal* published several studies showing a connection between polio, diphtheria, measles, tetanus, and smallpox vaccines and the development of multiple sclerosis several years later.[3]

More recently, concern arose about the correlation between the hepatitis B vaccination (HBV) and MS. An article in the *Annals of Pharmacotherapy* concludes that HBV is associated with multiple sclerosis, along with many other serious conditions.[4] This vaccine is now given to newborns before they leave the hospital; yet it is highly toxic to infants, whose blood-brain barriers and immune systems are not yet fully developed.

Stress

Stress is today's number-one "body breaker." Stress is the sum total of all the mental and physical input we encounter. When your capacity for input goes into overload, stress essentially becomes distress. Job pressures, relationship problems, health conditions, noise, pollution, financial concerns, and keeping up with the fast pace of life today all create distress. We all need some stress in our life to keep motivated and feel purposeful, but most of us are on overdrive physically, mentally, and emotionally, to the point of creating imbalance.

Those with MS usually have one thing in common—before they were diagnosed they had an extremely traumatic psychological event and/or high levels of chronic stress. Physical, emotional, and mental stress weaken your central nervous system.

How Chronic Stress Damages Your Body

The body has a parasympathetic and sympathetic nervous system. The parasympathetic dominates when you are at rest, breathing comfortably, and experiencing a normal heart rate. Sympathetic dominance is responsible for your fight-or-flight response. It puts you into action by flooding your body first with adrenaline and then with cortisol, which continues to be produced for hours afterward. Under healthy circumstances, both systems work together to keep the body in a state of homeostasis. However, in most people today the sympathetic mode is operating too much of the time, making it harder for the body to return to its resting state and creating chronic stress that could ultimately lead to adrenal exhaustion.

When the adrenals malfunction, the output of two of its hormones—cortisol and dehydroepiandrosterone (DHEA, an anti-aging hormone)—becomes imbalanced. The resulting abnormal ratio of cortisol to DHEA makes you feel exhausted. The high level of cortisol suppresses the activity of certain white blood cells, which compromises your immune system, impairs your endocrine (hormonal) system, and depletes nutrients, setting the stage for yeast, viruses, and bacterial infections to thrive. Free radicals (atoms that are highly reactive due to one or more unpaired electrons) become more abundant and cause oxidative stress, which damages cells. In MS patients this manifests as the destruction of brain cells and tissue, i.e., the myelin sheath.

Elevated cortisol to DHEA ratios also increase blood pressure, respiration, and heart rate; lower blood sugar and decrease insulin sensitivity; accelerate bone loss, fat accumulation, and muscle wasting; cause insomnia; and impair the body's ability to detoxify heavy metals. Most importantly, elevated cortisol lowers the levels of secretory IgA (mucosal antibodies), which protect the mucosal lining of the gut. When this barrier is weakened, yeasts, fungus, undigested food particles, and other antigens (foreign invaders) escape into the blood and lymph systems, creating an inflammatory response and compromising your immune system.

Acidic Body

For optimal health, your body needs to maintain a balance between acidity and alkalinity. The body's fluids and tissues have different optimal pH values. For example, the blood needs to be at a pH of 7.35 (slightly alkaline); saliva, between 6.4 and

6.8; and the large intestine, between 5.6 and 6.4.

Acidity is one of the main causes of inflammation because it disrupts body chemistry. Inflammatory antigens caused by acidity attack various parts of the body, including the myelin sheath, causing demyelination.

What are we exposed to in today's world that creates this acidity? Stress (resulting in hormonal imbalance), caffeine, alcohol, recreational drugs, pharmaceutical medications, tobacco, environmental chemicals, and unhealthy foods (refined sugars and carbohydrates, excess red meat, pasteurized dairy products, and processed foods). An acidic body leads to an inflamed and pained body, which over time becomes a diseased body.

The bloodstream must maintain an alkaline pH in the range of 7.35 to 7.45 at all times to sustain life. Your body has various mechanisms for maintaining that blood pH, as without this protective mechanism, death would result. However, when the body becomes acidic it can wreak havoc on your system. In order to maintain the proper pH it leaches calcium and other minerals (which are alkaline) from the rest of the body to buffer the acidity in the bloodstream and maintain an alkaline condition. Eventually bone loss, or osteoporosis, occurs. The longer this process goes unchecked, the greater the depletion of other minerals as well as proteins, causing an imbalance in body chemistry and the further deterioration of tissues, organs, joints, and bones. This depletion can go unnoticed for many years because blood tests will give "normal" results until an organ or system is in an exhausted state. Then you wonder why all of a sudden you have an autoimmune disease.

Trauma

It has been well documented in a number of cases that MS has erupted after people have experienced a physical trauma to the head or spinal column. Such injuries can be minor, such as a bump on the head, or severe, such as a serious fall or whiplash from a car accident. Whenever there is an injury, inflammation occurs as part of the body's natural healing response. However, when there is already an abundance of fungal toxins present in the body, the inflamed area becomes more vulnerable to them. Some believe that an injury to the head, neck, or spinal column may create a portal for toxins at the site to reach the central nervous system.

Poor Diet and Food Allergies

Diet alters your body chemistry either positively or negatively. A poor diet of refined sugars, gluten, alcohol, dairy, trans fats, and processed foods destroys cellular function and disrupts the ecology of your digestive system. In the next chapter I will discuss this in greater detail.

Poor digestion results from eating denatured foods and leads to proteins not being broken down properly. Undigested proteins putrefy in your gut and enter your bloodstream. Once these proteins leave the gut, they alert the immune system that antigens have entered your body. The immune system then begins producing protein antibodies to fight the invaders. Also in response, your body releases histamine. Your adrenal glands, which supply a natural antihistamine, weaken over time when this process is ongoing, as does your immune system function, and you become allergic not only to food, but also to environmental toxins.

Environmental Toxicity

Our polluted environment is another factor responsible for the body's tissues becoming saturated with toxicity. Heavy metals (aluminum, cadmium, lead, and mercury), pesticides, fungicides, GMOs, molds, and synthetic chemicals surround us. Our bodies absorb these toxins and cannot excrete them as fast as they enter. These toxins add to the burden of our immune system, which may already be under attack by digestive and microbial toxins.

Genetics

Your inherited genes may determine your strengths and weaknesses. However, it is my observation that one's phenotype (the observable physical or biochemical characteristics of an organism as determined by both genetic makeup and environmental/lifestyle influences) plays a more important role than genetics alone in determining which imbalances will surface. For example, a family history of MS would not necessarily lead to someone developing MS if he or she has a healthy diet and lifestyle.

CONCLUSION

Chronic inflammation and infection are the cause of MS and almost all disease. While the body's natural response to injury and infection is an inflammatory process that helps neutralize harmful microorganisms, such as when you scrape your knee, chronic inflammation produces free radicals that overwhelm the body's antioxidant defenses, causing untold damage.

Inflammation is the result of four factors: infections (candida, parasites, viruses, and bacteria); nutritional deficiency and toxicity; environmental toxicity; and unmanaged psychological stress. Some people with MS have excesses in all areas, whereas some have them magnified in one or two areas. What is consistent in all MS cases is the presence of candida over-growth. The variability of the above-mentioned factors and the fact that Western medicine ignores them as causes of MS account for the lack of success in treating the condition.

What you need to understand is that before you knew you had MS, it was at least ten to fifteen years in the making. The central nervous system is the slowest system in the body to heal, so patience and tenacity are a must. Looking for a magic bullet will only lead to disappointment and further decline. The best approach toward healing MS is to become educated, apply the protocols that feel right to you, and be committed to change your lifestyle for the better.

CHAPTER FOUR

POOR DIET: TRASH IN = TRASH OUT

THE IMPORTANCE OF DIET

We must eat not only to survive but also to sustain vitality and optimize the functioning of the more than 300 trillion cells that make up our bodies. The digestion of food—as it breaks down into vitamins, minerals, fatty acids, and glycerol—is a complex chemistry, and what we eat can alter that chemistry either positively or negatively. You are what you digest, absorb, utilize, and eliminate, so a healthy diet is one of the most important components to preventive health and to healing a diseased body. What you eat can either rebuild or weaken your immune system as well as determine the quality of your aging process.

The increasing numbers of people with allergies, diabetes, heart disease, mental illness, autoimmune diseases, and cancers can be attributed in part to having an unhealthy diet. As I've pointed out, the average American diet consists of large amounts of trans fats, refined sugar, refined carbohydrates, caffeine, alcohol, and processed foods that are filled with chemicals and preservatives. How can our cells thrive on artificial and depleted food? They can't.

The liver, which has more than five hundred functions, is your body's main detoxifier. When you eat a poor diet, your liver, lungs, skin, kidneys, and bowels must work that much harder to eliminate food toxins, chemicals, and preservatives, and to counter the assault of the environmental toxins that you encounter each day. What you eat is vital to keeping your body running smoothly and to easing the stress on your organs.

Chronic disease is directly related to being nutritionally deficient and toxic over a period of time. The most common symptom that my MS clients report is lack of energy. Fatigue is the result of a toxic and nutritionally deficient body. Signs of degeneration and deprivation set in slowly until the wake-up call is loud enough that you can no longer ignore your condition. At that point, though, your physician is likely to box you with a diagnosis that you feel you can never overcome, such as MS.

It's a mistake to think that junk food will not negatively affect every cell in your body. Your body will pay the price. The equation is very simple: trash in equals trash out. The great news is that you have control over the food choices you make. Once you educate yourself and examine your relationship to food, you can start to make the necessary modifications—and you'll quickly notice improvements.

THE IMPACT OF NUTRITION

With all of our money and technology, the United States is one of the sickest nations in comparison to the rest of the world. Our poor-quality diet of antibiotic- and hormone-laden meat and dairy products, trans fats, refined carbohydrates, and sugar is to blame.

Medical students receive hardly any instruction in nutrition as part of their four-year education. A 2006 survey of 106 universities found that, on the average, students received 24 hours of instruction. "Only 40 schools required the minimum 25 hours recommended by the National Academy of Sciences."[1] I consider this minimal requirement itself to be grossly inadequate. Clients tell me that their doctors say to them, "What you eat has nothing to do with your condition. Neither does taking vitamins." This couldn't be further from the truth.

There is also a general view in our society that says, "I'm going to die anyway, so what does it matter what I eat?" This viewpoint needs to be reexamined. It is true that all of us will pass over someday, but it is possible to age with quality and to retain our physical and mental agility, flexibility, and soundness as we do. Although you are more than your body, without it you do not exist. Anyone with MS knows how precious it is to have health. Making the choice to eat a healthy, balanced diet is one of the secrets of conquering MS.

THE MENTAL AND EMOTIONAL EFFECTS OF DIET

One of the most neglected factors regarding diet is how much it affects your nervous system and emotions. Poor diet can create depression, anxiety, and serious mental illness. A lack of B vitamins due to excess intake of refined carbohydrates and sugar disrupts neurotransmitters (chemical messengers of the nervous system) that help you to sleep and think rationally.

According to Gerald Ross, MD, "Food sensitivities, nutritional imbalances, and indoor air pollution can profoundly influence brain function."[2] The brain and the gut are interconnected, just as all systems in our body are. There is a direct correlation between the undigested food particles and toxins that pass through your gut and the toxicity that reaches your brain. These toxins cause not only physical symptoms but psychological ones as well—your emotions and thoughts are affected by what is going on in your brain, your gut, and your overall physiology. Therefore, healthy eating is as important to your mental and emotional health as it is to your physical well-being.

The canning and processing of foods depletes them of enzymes, vitamins, minerals, and micronutrients. Our grocery stores have been filled with aisles of dead food since World War II, when we first began canning and processing food for our soldiers. But that war ended more than a half century ago—it is time for you to educate yourself about how the depleted foods that are sold are assaulting your body.

THE MAIN OFFENDERS

It seems like almost every day we hear stories about this or that food not being good for you. While there are many theories about food and diet, some valid and some disputable, there is growing consensus that certain substances are detrimental and contribute to a compromised immune system.

Refined Sugar

Refined sugar in any of its forms (sucrose, high fructose corn syrup, dextrose, etc.) is one of the most harmful substances you can consume. It has absolutely no nutritional value, depletes the vital vitamins and minerals that you need to sustain yourself, and wreaks havoc with your immune system and pancreas (which regulates your blood-sugar levels). Well-known nutritionist Ann Louise Gittleman states: "There are over sixty ailments that have been associated with sugar consumption in medical literature."[3] Cancer, *Candida albicans*, and human immunodeficiency virus (HIV) all thrive on sugar.

Exacerbations of MS symptoms worsen and become more frequent when patients ingest high-sugar foods because sugar upsets the body chemistry, causing an inflammatory response and weakening the immune system. According to Ray C. Wunderlich, MD, and Dwight K. Kalita, PhD, "The ingestion of large amounts of sugar paralyzes the phagocytic capacity of our white blood cells."[4] This means your white blood cells, which play a major role in the functioning of a strong immune system, cannot identify and destroy foreign invaders. Over time, this incapacity opens the door for more imbalances and disease in the body.

When you begin to read labels, you will see that almost every processed food on the market—from canned goods to breads to salt—contains sugar in some form. Refined sugar is disguised as sucrose, fructose, dextrose, brown sugar, glucose, evaporated cane juice, high-fructose corn syrup, lactose, and maltose. Don't be misled if the label says "organic cane sugar." This, as well as agave and honey, will have a detrimental effect when you're trying to rid your body of candida.

The United States is a nation addicted to sugar. In 1890, the average American ate 10 pounds of sugar a year. Today, that figure is over 150 pounds.

Unfortunately, in our society sugar is not just something that tastes good. It has also become an emotional pacifier. Refined sugar may satisfy your psychological needs for a moment, but ultimately it will destroy your body. The most important step you can take to stop the progression of your MS is to get the refined sugar out of your diet (see Table 4.1).

TABLE 4.1 Fifty-nine Reasons Why Sugar Ruins Your Health

1. Sugar can suppress the immune system.
2. Sugar upsets the minerals in the body.
3. Sugar may cause hyperacidity, anxiety, difficulty concentrating, and crankiness in children.
4. Sugar produces a significant rise in triglycerides.
5. Sugar contributes to the reduction of the body's defense against bacterial infection.
6. Sugar can cause kidney damage.
7. Sugar reduces high-density lipoproteins (HDL).
8. Sugar leads to chromium deficiency.
9. Sugar can lead to cancer of the breast, ovaries, intestines, prostate, or rectum.
10. Sugar increases fasting levels of glucose and insulin.
11. Sugar causes copper deficiency.
12. Sugar interferes with absorption of calcium and magnesium.
13. Sugar can weaken eyesight.
14. Sugar raises the level of neurotransmitters called serotonin.
15. Sugar can cause hypoglycemia.
16. Sugar can produce an acidic stomach.
17. Sugar can raise adrenaline levels in children.
18. Sugar malabsorption is frequent in patients with functional bowel disease.
19. Sugar can cause signs of premature aging.
20. Sugar can lead to alcoholism.
21. Sugar leads to tooth decay.
22. Sugar contributes to obesity.
23. High intake of sugar increases the risk of Crohn's Disease and ulcerative colitis.
24. Sugar can cause symptoms often found in people with gastric and duodenal ulcers.
25. Sugar can lead to arthritis.
26. Sugar can contribute to asthma.
27. Sugar can cause *Candida albicans* (yeast infection).
28. Sugar can contribute to gallstones.
29. Sugar can lead to heart disease.

TABLE 4.1 *(continued)*

30. Sugar can cause appendicitis.
31. Sugar can lead to multiple sclerosis.
32. Sugar can cause hemorrhoids.
33. Sugar can contribute to varicose veins.
34. Sugar can elevate glucose and insulin responses in oral contraceptive users.
35. Sugar can lead to periodontal disease.
36. Sugar can contribute to osteoporosis.
37. Sugar contributes to salivary acidity.
38. Sugar can cause a decrease in insulin sensitivity.
39. Sugar leads to decreased glucose tolerance.
40. Sugar can decrease growth hormones.
41. Sugar can increase cholesterol.
42. Sugar can increase the systolic blood pressure.
43. Sugar can cause drowsiness and decreased activity in children.
44. Sugar can cause migraine headaches.
45. Sugar can interfere with absorption of protein.
46. Sugar can cause food allergies.
47. Sugar can contribute to diabetes.
48. Sugar can cause toxemia during pregnancy.
49. Sugar can contribute to eczema in children.
50. Sugar can lead to cardiovascular disease.
51. Sugar can impair the structure of DNA.
52. Sugar can change the structure of proteins.
53. Sugar can contribute to sagging skin by changing the structure of collagen.
54. Sugar can lead to cataracts.
55. Sugar can cause emphysema.
56. Sugar can cause atherosclerosis.
57. Sugar can promote an elevation of low-density proteins (LDL).
58. Sugar can cause free radicals in the bloodstream.
59. Sugar lowers the enzymes' ability to function.

Source: Nancy Appleton, PhD, *Lick the Sugar Habit* (Avery Publishing Group, 1996). Used with permission.

Trans Fats (bad fats)

The United States is finally recognizing that trans fats, which have already been banned in Denmark and Canada, are major contributors to heart disease and other serious health conditions. Any food that lists "partially hydrogenated" or "hydrogenated" oil among its ingredients contains trans fats. This means that the oil has been heated to a high temperature for the sole reason of preserving the food product for a longer shelf life.

Trans fats are found in pastries, breads, crackers, processed foods, microwave popcorn, chips, cookies, and margarines. Research has shown that margarines with trans fats—not butter—are the real cause of blocked arteries. These bad fats are poison to anyone with MS because they set off an inflammatory response in the body.

Refined Carbohydrates

I call refined carbohydrates—such as white flour, white rice, and refined grains—"glue and goo." These foods include pastries, cookies, muffins, bagels, breads, donuts, and crackers. Refined carbohydrates create mucus that coats the lining of your GI tract, which interferes with the processes of absorbing nutrients and eliminating waste. They are irritants that weaken the intestinal walls, contributing to leaky gut syndrome and ultimately leading to inflammation, allergies, candida, celiac disease, and malnutrition.

The packaging on many breads that contain refined flour (whether white or wheat) states that they have been enriched with vitamins and minerals, meaning that they have been added back into the bread. The truth is that when the flour is bleached and refined it loses important micronutrients—fiber in particular—which are still lacking after enrichment. Fiber is essential for proper elimination and for keeping your blood cholesterol levels down.

Because refined carbohydrates convert rapidly to glucose (sugar), they contribute to the alarming rates of people with constipation, irritable bowel syndrome, and imbalances in blood-sugar levels, which can lead to both hypoglycemia (low blood sugar) and diabetes. Also, the bleaching agent used in refined flour, nitrogen trichloride, is poisonous and has been linked to ulcers, schizophrenia, and MS.

Dairy Products

Bovine dairy products (those from cows) are the leading cause of food allergies. Allergies to these products cause sinus problems and gastrointestinal complaints such as gas, bloating, cramps, and diarrhea. Hyperactivity and irritability are common reactions, especially in children. Asthma, headaches, joint and muscle pain, depression, lack of energy, and skin problems are also attributed to dairy allergies.

Lactaid milk, in which the lactose (milk sugar) has been removed, was created to help those who are lactose intolerant. However, this doesn't solve the problem for everyone who has trouble with milk. There's a difference between being lactose intolerant and having a milk allergy, and most people who can't drink milk have both conditions. Lactose intolerance means that you lack the enzyme that breaks down lactose. Having a milk allergy means that the body is unable to recognize the milk protein, sees it as a foreign invader, and defends itself by creating an allergic response.

Many in the medical community and advertising industry tell us that drinking milk is the best way to get calcium. Women are especially targeted because of the rising levels of osteoporosis in our country. Yet the fact is that only 30 percent of the calcium in eight ounces of milk is actually absorbed by the body. Pasteurization destroys the enzyme phosphatase. Without phosphatase our bodies cannot use phosphorous, and without phosphorous we cannot assimilate calcium.

Think about it—we're the only species that drinks milk from another species. How do cows get their calcium? Not by drinking milk from another species, but by eating grass (if they're being raised humanely). Plant foods such as sesame seeds, almonds, broccoli, carrots, and dark-green leafy vegetables are high in calcium—higher in some cases than cow's milk. These also contain trace minerals that assist the calcium to enter your bones.

The real cause of calcium deficiencies—and osteoporosis—is excessive consumption of high-acid foods, such as animal meats, caffeine, refined carbohydrates and sugars, and pasteurized milk and dairy products. Pasteurization and homogenization of cow's milk alter its mineral composition, making it acidic to the body. Consumption of these foods forces the body to leach calcium and other minerals from the bones to buffer the acidity in the bloodstream, which, as mentioned earlier, must maintain an alkaline condition of pH 7.35. To maintain that pH level, the blood robs minerals from the body's biggest storehouse of minerals, the musculoskeletal system. In short, consuming dairy products creates exactly the opposite effect that you may be trying to achieve.

Antibiotics and Hormones in Dairy Products

The major factor you need to consider when deciding whether to ingest dairy products is the use of antibiotics and hormones in raising cows. According to a *Newsweek* article, "Milk is allowed to contain a certain concentration of eighty different antibiotics—all used in dairy cows to prevent udder infections. With every glassful, people swallow a minute amount of several antibiotics."[5] Bovine growth hormone (RBGH), which was produced through gene splicing to increase milk production, also ends up in the milk. These hormones and antibiotics, which are permitted by the government, are creating imbalances in our children and adults.

I'm not talking only about milk, but also about products made from milk, such as cheese, ice cream, sour cream, and yogurt. The American Dairy Association is spending big bucks to convince you that "Milk does a body good," as the billboard says, but I ask you to think again.

Animal Protein

Animal proteins, such as red meat, pork, chicken, turkey, and fish, are also questionable food sources for a variety of reasons. Pork, beef, chicken, and turkey that are not from organically raised animals also contain antibiotics and hormones. These are passed on to consumers and cause hormonal and yeast imbalances.

Pork contains higher concentrations of parasites because of what pigs are fed and the fact that they do not eliminate toxins efficiently. Red meat is more acidic to your body chemistry than chicken and turkey, especially when cooked beyond medium-rare and when eaten with grains or starchy vegetables such as potatoes. So organically raised chicken and turkey are better choices. The acidity from heavy meat eating adds to inflammation and makes MS symptoms worse.

Unfortunately, fish also contain toxins because our oceans have become polluted with heavy metals and chemicals. Shellfish are particularly high in contaminants, as they are bottom feeders and absorb higher concentrations of chemicals and mercury. Stay away from all tuna since the mercury levels are very high. Fish such as wild-caught Pacific salmon and cod are high in essential fatty acids, which help to restore the myelin sheath, so there are advantages to eating them. However, finding clean sources can be a challenge (see Note, page 251).

Caffeine

Caffeine—whether in the form of coffee, energy drinks (e.g., Red Bull), soda, tea, or chocolate—is acidic and raises blood-sugar levels. It also stimulates the adrenal glands to release hormones that put the body into an adrenaline-rush response, increasing the heart rate. The body responds by releasing stored sugar, which causes the pancreas to kick out insulin to bring sugar levels back into balance. Overconsumption of caffeine perpetuates this cycle, exhausting the adrenals and the pancreas, whose health we depend on for optimal energy. This rise in sugar feeds candida overgrowth in the body.

In addition, the excessive acidity from caffeinated products irritates your nervous system and creates inflammation, bringing pain and destruction to your myelin sheath.

Alcohol

All alcohol is a neurotoxin and goes directly into the bloodstream, creating an inflammatory response and depleting vitamins and minerals in your body. Wine, beer, champagne, and sake do more damage to the body than distilled alcohol, such as vodka, because they are higher in sugar, which increases blood-sugar levels and feeds candida. For anyone with MS, consuming alcohol is a sure-fire way to accelerate the degeneration of your central nervous system.

Food Allergens

Food allergies arise when there are imbalances in your gut, such as maldigestion from eating refined, depleted, and processed food. Large quantities of undigested food particles irritating and passing through the lining of the GI tract will cause an allergic reaction in the bloodstream. The most common food allergies are to milk, corn, soy, citrus fruits, chocolate, eggs, nightshade vegetables (eggplant, peppers, potatoes, tomatoes), and gluten. Allergies to even healthy foods, such as certain fruits and nuts, can also arise when your digestive system is out of balance.

Gluten intolerance and celiac disease are increasing at alarming rates, and people with MS need to pay special attention to these conditions. A study published in the *Lancet* states that *Candida albicans* may act as a trigger in the onset of celiac disease in those who are genetically susceptible. There is a protein in *Candida albicans* known as HWP1, whose structure is similar to that of gluten. When a candida infection is present in the gut it can set off an immune system reaction to HWP1, which in turn causes an allergic reaction to gluten.[6]

Several medical researchers have examined the link between gluten sensitivity and neurodegenerative conditions. In a *Lancet Neurology* article entitled "Gluten Sensitivity: From Gut to Brain," Dr. Marios Hadjivassiliou and his colleagues state: "Gluten sensitivity is a systemic autoimmune disease with diverse manifestations. This disorder is characterised by abnormal immunological responsiveness to ingested gluten in genetically susceptible individuals. Coeliac disease, or gluten-sensitive enteropathy, is only one aspect of a range of possible manifestations of gluten sensitivity. Although neurological manifestations in patients with established coeliac disease have been reported since 1966, it was not until thirty years later that, in some individuals, gluten sensitivity was shown to manifest solely with neurological dysfunction."[7] Part of their study revealed a segment of patients who had white matter lesions on the brain or spinal cord that were similar to those found in patients with multiple sclerosis.

White flour, rye, oats (due to cross-contamination), barley, spelt, kamut, triticale, and wheat contain gluten, a protein that is abrasive to the GI tract and can strip the villi. These hair-like projections attached to the intestinal walls help to absorb nutrients and keep the gut clean of yeast and bacteria. In addition, wheat has been hybridized and is subject to a process known as gluten deamidation, in which it is converted to wheat isolates. These are used as binders and emulsifiers in foods, including meat products, sauces, soups, and some beverages. The isolates are more detrimental than the gluten in native wheat and can cause major disruptions in the body.

If you want to know whether you are gluten intolerant and/or are having autoimmune responses, you can contact Cyrex Laboratories (Cyrexlabs.com). Their Antibody Array 3 tests your transglutaminase reactivity, and their Antibody Array 4 lets you know if you have cross-reactivity to foods other than just gluten. There is a strong relationship between transglutaminases (enzymes) testing positive and autoimmune responses. Those who test positive for transglutaminase and/or celiac disease must avoid gluten permanently.

Soy is another food that has been a topic for debate. In America, the market is flooded with genetically modified soy protein foods, processed tofu, and soy protein powders, which may be harmful to your body, as some research has shown. However, if you examine the diets of Asians, you will find that they use fermented soy products, such as miso and tempeh, and in small amounts. Soy in these forms is more digestible and high in essential amino acids and B vitamins. Unfortunately, fermented soy products are not allowed on a candida-cure diet because they can aggravate candida. The only allowable soy on my program is Bragg Liquid Aminos because the soy is unfermented and non-GMO.

A lot of people are allergic to soy and experience gas and bloating when they eat it. If you have this reaction, I recommend avoiding soy products. There are also studies that say large amounts of soy protein can disrupt thyroid function. Because the jury is still out on whether soy is good or bad for you, I feel it is best to stay away from it.

Artificial Sweeteners and Sugar Alcohols

Artificial sweeteners, such as aspartame, acesulfame-K, saccharin, and sucralose, are promoted as an alternative to sugar for people who want to lose weight or eliminate sugar from their diets. But diet sodas and food products that contain these artificial sweeteners are very damaging to the body. The chemicals used to create these sweeteners, or to change the molecular structure of sugar to create them, are known carcinogens. Aspartame, a known neurotoxin, has been linked to neurological symptoms and conditions such as blurred vision, headaches, dizziness, memory loss, numbness, MS, ALS, and Parkinson's disease.

Sugar alcohols, such as erythritol, maltitol, mannitol, sorbitol, and xylitol, are rising in popularity because they are not as damaging to the body as artificial sweeteners. Sugar alcohols are neither sugars nor alcohols. They are carbohydrates with a chemical structure that partially resembles sugar and partially resembles alcohol, but they don't contain ethanol as do alcoholic beverages. They are incompletely absorbed and metabolized by the body and consequently contribute fewer calories than most sugars; however, because they are not fully absorbed they can ferment in the intestines and cause bloating, gas, and diarrhea.

Of the sugar alcohols listed above, I prefer xylitol in small quantities because it is made by our bodies in the metabolism of carbohydrates, it raises oral pH to be more alkaline when ingested, and it is antimicrobial. Commercial xylitol is obtained from corn or the bark of birch trees. I prefer the latter to avoid products made with genetically modified corn. I suggest taking it only in small amounts (under 1 teaspoon, not daily) for two reasons. Xylitol is a carbohydrate, which means it will feed candida if used in large quantities, and although it is obtained from a natural source, it is chemically processed. Any artificial sweetener or sugar alcohol consumed in moderate to large quantities is toxic to the body.

SUPPLEMENTATION

In today's world, a good diet by itself cannot keep your body healthy, let alone heal MS. Along with a healthy diet, your body requires supplementation. Because modern agricultural practices have depleted our soil, we must eat five to ten times the amount our grandparents ate to obtain the same nutrient value. More than ever before, our bodies must also cope with greater environmental toxicity from pesticides, herbicides, fungicides, genetically modified seeds, heavy metals, and synthetic chemicals. On top of that, increased stress levels have weakened our bodies, making supplementation necessary to offset the imbalance. In Part Four you will learn how to decide which supplements are right for you.

WATER

Last but not least is the topic of water. Our society is dehydrated and, as the eminent researcher F. Batmanghelidj stated, "dehydration is the number one stressor of the human body—or *any* living matter."[8]

How can you keep your body running smoothly when it's made up of 80 percent water and you drink fewer than eight cups of water a day? You can't. When you do, your "plumbing" gets backed up—your lymphatic system becomes sluggish, your kidneys become overstressed, your colon becomes constipated, and your liver and gallbladder become congested. Autotoxicity sets in as you reabsorb the toxins that your body is unable to eliminate through these channels, creating an environment that promotes autoimmune diseases and cancer.

In Chapter 10 I will discuss the key elements for nourishing your body with foods and drinks that will support a healthy immune system.

CHAPTER FIVE

THE DIGESTIVE SYSTEM AND IMMUNITY

THE SEEDS OF DISEASE

One of the most overlooked systems in the body is the digestive system. Yet an imbalance in this system—comprised of the mouth, salivary glands, stomach, pancreas, liver, gallbladder, and small and large intestines—is responsible for the onset of most chronic progressive and autoimmune diseases. As naturopath Mark Percival states in *Functional Dietetics*, "Destructive eating habits lead first to gastrointestinal dysfunction and then subsequently contribute to virtually every noninfectious disease known to us (and likely some of the infectious diseases as well)."[1]

While there has been a lot of attention focused these days on the importance of a healthy immune system, few people realize that about 75 percent of the immune system's cells are produced in the digestive tract. Scientists tell us that there are ten times more bacterial cells living inside the GI tract, the stomach, and intestines than there are human cells in the entire body. The small and large intestines have a combined length of twenty to twenty-five feet, the width of a tennis court if you were to stretch them out.

A balanced ecosystem in the GI tract has a ratio of 85 percent healthy microorganisms to 15 percent unhealthy ones. Inadequate diets based on foods that are depleted of nutrients and filled with chemicals and preservatives upset this ratio and can create maldigestion, malabsorption, intestinal dysbiosis (overgrowth of microbes such as fungi, parasites, bacteria, and viruses), and elimination problems. What's more, these problems are not isolated conditions that affect just the digestive system; they also affect other systems of your body, including the immune system (see Figure 5.1).

MALDIGESTION

Chronic poor diet contributes to maldigestion, which occurs when the body is unable to properly break down food. Reasons for this include lack of hydrochloric acid (HCl) in the stomach, inadequate chewing, poor food combining, drinking excessive liquids with meals, pancreatic enzyme deficiencies, hiatal hernia, and stress.

When food goes undigested, the particles and their toxic by-products become intestinal irritants that can cross the mucosal lining of the stomach and enter the bloodstream (leaky gut syndrome). The blood sees these particles as foreign invaders and creates an antibody response by having the white blood cells come to the rescue to defend your body. However, this activity produces inflammation, allergic reactions, and food sensitivities. In addition, the undigested food particles produce fermentation, which fuels fungal overgrowth and the proliferation of bacteria and parasites. Symptoms of maldigestion include belching, bloating, gas, abdominal pain, and heartburn.

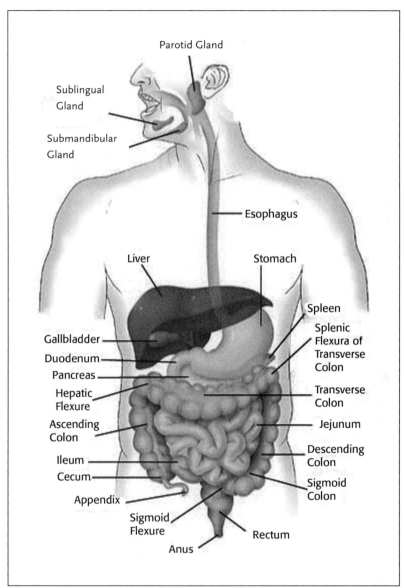

Figure 5.1 Anatomy of the Digestive System

ENZYME DEFICIENCIES

Enzyme deficiencies are a major contributor to maldigestion. Enzymes are proteins that act as catalysts to ignite chemical reactions in the body. While the body does manufacture its own enzymes, it must also make use of those in food to have optimal health. Most enzymes are destroyed in foods that are processed, refined, or cooked at temperatures above 118 degrees Fahrenheit. Raw or lightly steamed foods, on the other hand, are rich in enzymes.

When enzymes are lacking in the body, the pancreas, which secretes digestive enzymes, takes on a greater load. The pancreas also has the job of producing insulin, the hormone that maintains blood-sugar levels. Therefore diets loaded with refined carbohydrates, sugar, and cooked and processed foods overwork the pancreas and weaken its performance, making us more susceptible to yeast overgrowth and conditions like hypoglycemia and diabetes.

MALABSORPTION

Malabsorption occurs when the uptake of food from the intestines is impaired. Without proper absorption, you cannot nourish your cells and they begin to degenerate. Nutrients are absorbed from food by the villi (the hair-like projections lining the intestines), but a poor diet and toxic overload in the body can strip the villi and inhibit their function, creating malabsorption.

The main causes of malabsorption are maldigestion and microbial overgrowth (bacteria, fungi, parasites, worms, and viruses). Common symptoms of malabsorption are fatigue, thinning hair, dry skin, depression, susceptibility to bruising, unexplainable weight loss, and constipation or diarrhea.

DYSBIOSIS

Intestinal dysbiosis results from an imbalance of microorganisms (yeast, bacteria, parasites, and viruses), which upsets the digestive system and interferes with nutrient absorption. Dysbiosis is caused by poor diet; alcohol; recreational drugs; stress; maldigestion; elimination problems; the overuse of antibiotics; steroids such as cortisone, prednisone, and birth control pills; nonsteroidal anti-inflammatory drugs (NSAIDs); heavy metal toxins; and immunosuppressive drugs.

When unhealthy microorganisms take over the gut, your immune system is put under constant stress to defend your body from these infections. Intestinal dysbiosis is a contributing cause in rheumatoid arthritis, MS, vitamin B12 deficiency, chronic fatigue, cystic acne, the early stages of colon and breast cancer, eczema, food allergies and sensitivities, inflammatory bowel disease, irritable bowel syndrome, psoriasis, Sjögren's syndrome (a postmenopausal immunological disorder), and steatorrhea (excess fat in the stools). The most common form of intestinal dysbiosis is *Candida albicans* overgrowth.

LEAKY GUT SYNDROME

Maldigestion, malabsorption, and intestinal dysbiosis set the stage for leaky gut syndrome. As I've discussed, leaky gut is a condition in which the intestines' mucosal lining becomes irritated, inflamed, and more porous. This allows undigested food particles and microorganisms and their by-products to pass through the lining into the bloodstream. Candida overgrowth, NSAIDs, poor diet, heavy metals, daily aspirin use, and gluten sensitivity (to wheat, rye, barley, white flour, spelt, kamut, and oats) all contribute to irritating the lining.

"Leaky gut triggers a state of continuous and prolonged stress in and on the immune system," says Dr. Jeffrey S. Bland.[2] Allergies are one of the first conditions to occur when someone has leaky gut. Other more serious conditions may follow.

The gut lining acts as a protective mucosal barrier and is your first line of defense to prevent infection. When pathogens and foreign organisms come into contact with the mucosal barrier, immune cells inside the gut produce secretory immunoglobin A (SigA), an antibody that attacks them. However, chronic stress continually suppresses SigA production and thus allows pathogens to enter your bloodstream and eventually to migrate to your brain and other tissues.

An article published in the *Annals of the New York Academy of Sciences* states: "There is growing evidence that increased intestinal permeability plays a pathogenic role in various autoimmune diseases including CD [celiac disease] and T1D [type 1 diabetes]. Therefore, we hypothesize that besides genetic and environmental factors, loss of intestinal barrier function is necessary to develop autoimmunity."[3]

Over time, the presence of bacteria, yeast/fungi, parasites, and viruses traveling in the bloodstream means that the body is under siege. As these toxins circulate in the bloodstream, organs such as the liver, the lymph glands, the brain, the lungs, and the kidneys become overloaded. When cellular communication is disrupted, cross-wiring of the RNA and DNA and the replication of unhealthy cells result, leading to autoimmune diseases and cancer. Simply put, leaky gut causes chronic inflammation, which eventually translates to chronic immune dysfunction as seen in MS. Your genetic predispositions will determine which organs and systems are affected.

LEAKY GUT AND THE LIVER

The liver is an amazing organ. The largest in the body, it has more than five hundred functions. You can't live without your liver. It assists with metabolism, storing vitamins and minerals, and detoxifying toxic compounds.

Here's just a small piece of the picture. The portal vein delivers blood from the small intestine to the liver containing not only nutrients from digested food, but also toxins. The nutrients are carried through the circulatory system to feed every cell of your body. But what happens to the toxins?

One of the liver's many tasks is to recognize and neutralize these poisons, which come from substances such as heavy metals, pesticides, toxic foods, alcohol, cigarettes, synthetic chemicals, medications, and the by-products of stress hormones. Leaky gut makes the job of the liver more difficult by forcing it to break down undigested proteins as well as deal with the microbes and their by-products that have entered it through the blood. If the liver can't keep up with the overload of toxins, they will be stored in the liver or recirculated in the body. The combined effect is an interference with the liver's efficiency.

The liver produces and secretes bile, which is stored in the gallbladder until it is needed by the small intestine to assist with fat digestion. In addition to breaking down fats and its other important roles, bile has antibacterial properties that help protect the small intestine from harmful bacteria, yeast, and parasites. However, in a toxic body bile often becomes thick and sludgy, hampering its flow and function. One result is that yeast, viruses, and bacteria flourish, upsetting the ratio of good to bad bacteria.

The function of bile can be compromised by an excess of estrogen hormones, which reduces bile flow and elevates bile cholesterol levels. This poses a risk of gallstones and the recirculation of estrogens, increasing the risk of cancers of the breast, ovaries, uterus, and prostate. People with MS need to be aware that imbalanced hormones are common in their condition.

An impaired liver can lead to problems in another area relevant to MS sufferers. An article in the journal *Lancet* states: "When the gut becomes leaky, more toxic substances are delivered to the liver, and if the liver's functional ability to detoxify is impaired, more metabolically active substances are delivered through the bloodstream to other tissues, including the brain."[4]

Like the GI tract lining, the blood-brain barrier can become compromised. When this happens, toxins that escape the liver become stored in fatty tissues, such as the cells of the brain and the central nervous system, causing inflammation and oxidative stress. This accounts for the wide range of noninfectious diseases you see today, specifically MS. Therefore, detoxifying the liver and gut is essential if you want to keep inflammatory agents out of the rest of your body.

ELIMINATION

The importance of elimination to overall health is grossly neglected by most doctors. Many people tell me that their doctors have said that daily bowel movements aren't necessary. This is false. Daily elimination is essential, and two to three movements a day is best.

The optimal transit time for food to go from your mouth out through your rectum is twenty-four hours. Yet in all my years of practice, I have found that the majority of people have transit times that range between forty-eight and seventy-four hours.

Looking at this on a larger scale, we see a nation that is suffering from an epidemic of constipation, irritable bowel syndrome, and colitis. The main cause of all these conditions is inadequate water and fiber intake from fresh fruits, vegetables, and whole grains. When grains are refined, both minerals and fiber are stripped away, robbing the body of nourishment and the assistance the fiber provides in cleaning the colon walls.

If your bowels are backed up, your GI tract must focus more on getting rid of waste than on absorbing nutrients, making you more vulnerable to malnutrition and dysbiosis. Elimination problems also cause autotoxicity. Toxins that are not released from your body fast enough are reabsorbed into the bloodstream. Constipation can also make the pH level in the large intestine more alkaline, which creates a breeding environment in which yeasts/fungi, parasites, bacteria, and viruses thrive.

THE IMMUNE SYSTEM

The last but most important area affected by an imbalance in the digestive system is the immune system, which is simply your body's mechanism for identifying self (what naturally belongs in the body) from non-self (foreign material) and using antigens to destroy or neutralize whatever is foreign (see Figure 5.2).

The immune system is composed of lymphocytes (B and T cells), the thymus, the spleen, the bone marrow, the lymph

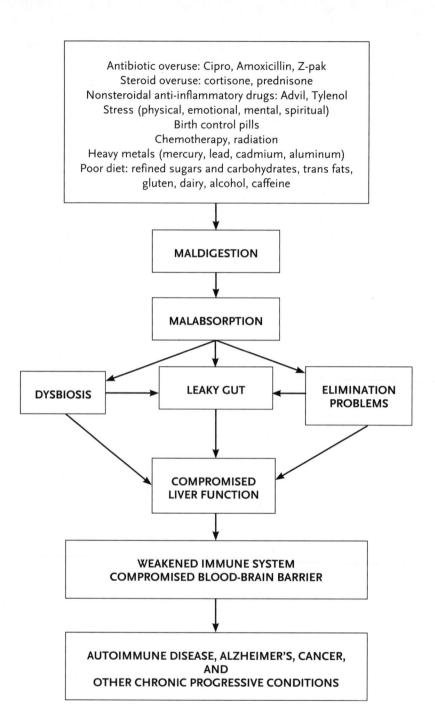

Figure 5.2: Digestive Tract and Immunity

nodes, the tonsils, the adenoids, the appendix, the lymphatic vessels, the liver, and Peyer's patches (clumps of lymphoid tissue in the small intestine). This gallant army of organs and cells comes to your rescue whenever foreign invaders attack your body. However, the immune system becomes weakened from chronic maldigestion, malabsorption, leaky gut, intestinal dysbiosis, elimination problems, compromised liver function, heavy metals, medications, stress hormones, and poor diet. This is why a toxic body can give rise to autoimmune diseases in which immune cells, such as the T cells, B cells, and macrophages, mistakenly attack the body's own tissues.

ALL BODY SYSTEMS ARE CONNECTED

You can now understand from what you've read in this chapter that every organ and system in your body is interconnected. All the systems "talk" to each other. If one organ becomes compromised, another organ will take over and try to compensate. When your gut is leaky, it fills your bloodstream with toxins. A polluted bloodstream and lymph system compromise your immune system. And an overtaxed immune system allows chronic inflammatory agents to enter your brain, heart, joints, muscles, organs, and so on.

MS is one of the conditions caused by an immune system that can't keep up with accumulated stressors. The key, then, is to keep toxins moving out faster than they accumulate so that the body can heal and stay balanced.

CHAPTER SIX

ENVIRONMENTAL TOXICITY

Although industrialization and technology have created many conveniences, your body is paying the price from exposure to an excessive amount of synthetic chemicals, heavy metals, electromagnetic frequencies, pesticides, and herbicides. Over time, this accumulation of environmental toxins can become a disease factor, contributing to conditions such as MS and other autoimmune diseases, allergies, asthma, attention deficit disorder (ADD), cancers, Alzheimer's disease, and Parkinson's disease, to name just a few.

CHEMICAL POLLUTION

Chemicals such as formaldehyde, dioxins, benzenes, asbestos, and carbon monoxide place a tremendous stress upon the body. There are thousands of chemicals produced in North America alone, many of which are used in our food in the form of preservatives, flavorings, and emulsifiers, as well as in the food processing industry. These chemicals are not visible to the naked eye, yet we are constantly exposed to them.

Most Americans store between 400 and 800 chemicals in their bodies, typically in fat cells, including those in the brain, whose fat content is approximately 60 percent. This is of special concern for those afflicted with MS. Over 200 chemicals are found in a newborn's umbilical cord blood.

One study cited a U.S. Environmental Protection Agency (EPA) estimate, stating that "1.5 trillion gallons of pollutants leak into the ground each year, with the highest incidence of contaminants from lead, nitrates (from fertilizers), and radon. Over 700 chemicals have been found in tap water, but testing is done on less than 200 of these."[1] The EPA's Office of Toxic Substances reported in 1989 that 551,034,696 pounds of industrial chemicals had been dumped into public sewage storage. The total amount of air emissions pumped into the atmosphere was 2,427,061,906 pounds. They estimated that a grand total of 5,705,670,380 pounds of chemical pollutants had been released into the environment in that same year.[2] These numbers are high enough to make anyone sick, and that was over twenty years ago.

INDOOR POLLUTION

One of the major health hazards that environmental and health organizations are concerned about is indoor health pollution. Advances in technology have allowed us to build more energy-efficient buildings and homes, but at the same time we have also created "sick building syndrome," meaning that chemicals and pollutants stay trapped inside buildings and houses. In 1998, an article in *Scientific American* stated that inhaling the chemical vapors from new carpet is equal to smoking three cigarettes a day.[3] Dr. Gerald Ross, the former president of the American Academy of Environmental Medicine, said, "Indoor air pollution can have profound effects on brain function."[4]

Polyvinyl Chloride (PVC), a plastic used in water-resistant products, vinyl flooring, wall coverings, and building materials, including newer residential plumbing pipes, is highly toxic and can leach into your drinking water. Dust mites, molds, fumes from common cleaning products, and petroleum pollutants from lubricants in personal-care and workshop products can also suppress your immune system.

GENETICALLY ALTERED FOOD

If you live in the United States, in addition to your food being treated with synthetic fertilizers, fungicides, and pesticides, much of it is genetically modified. Genetically modified organisms (GMOs) have had their genetic material altered to create characteristics that are not native to the plant or animal. The top genetically modified (GM) foods are soybeans, corn, canola, cottonseed, sugar beets, tomatoes, potatoes, rice, salmon, papaya, sprouts, squash, and animal feed. With livestock and fish being fed products containing GMOs, it is virtually impossible to avoid consuming them.

The government claims that producing genetically modified food will produce better crops and end world starvation. The truth is that chemical companies are managing this biotechnology and selling their seeds to farmers and making a profit. These GM crops have had their DNA altered to make them more pest and chemical resistant, but not only have the crops become more resistant; so have the weeds. "Superweeds" are now springing up in their place, requiring farmers to buy and apply even more deadly herbicides to deal with them. Thus, money making and greed motivate the drive to bring genetically modified food into our markets. These same chemical companies also produce pharmaceuticals.

We already know that pesticides and herbicides are toxic to the body, but the full effects of genetically modified food have not yet been fully disclosed. Studies are starting to surface showing that allergies, birth defects, cancer, degenerative diseases, superviruses, infertility in females and males, and weakened immune systems are connected to ingesting GM foods.[5]

Even though fifty countries around the world require genetically modified foods to be labeled, as of this writing the United States government still refuses to enforce mandatory labeling. The companies who manufacture the genetically modified seeds, pesticides, and herbicides would stand to lose a lot of money, and they have spent millions of dollars to defeat initiatives requiring them to label these products.

TAP AND BOTTLED WATER

As I mentioned above, our water supplies are contaminated with bacteria and chemicals. Contaminants in our water include microbial agents such as bacteria, viruses, and parasites; inorganic contaminants such as salts and metals from oil and gas production, mining, farming, and industrial and domestic wastewater discharging; pesticides, herbicides, and nitrates from agricultural and other sources; organic chemicals from industrial processing and petroleum production; and radioactive contaminants from oil, mining, and gas production—not to mention numerous other toxic substances.

Chlorine, used to "purify" water supplies by killing bacteria, is also toxic to our bodies. Fluoride is added to protect teeth and bones, but more and more research is showing that it is harmful, potentially even causing brain damage. Since bottled water has no strict regulations, we don't know what we are getting unless we use our own filtration systems.

MOLDS AND FUNGUS

More than 400 species of yeasts and molds can attack our bodies. Some are airborne as spores in the air that we breathe, and some live on the contaminated food that we eat. Among the most common are cryptococcosis, aspergillus (found on corn, wheat, and cheese), fusarium (found on bananas), dermatophytosis, histoplasmosis, penicillium (used in the antibiotic penicillin), diplodia, claviceps, and stachybotyrs. Mold can also be a problem in homes in basements, crawl spaces, walls, and other places where water accumulation or damage has occurred.

XENOESTROGENS

Many synthetic chemicals, pesticides, and herbicides are xenoestrogens; that is, they mimic estrogens. Phthalates, for example, are chemicals used to soften plastics and increase the life of fragrances. Bisphenol-A (BPA) is also used to make plastic products, including baby bottles, water bottles, and numerous other products for children and adults. Both of these substances have estrogen-like properties and negatively affect both women and men. Endometriosis and breast and uterine cancers have been attributed to xenoestrogens. For men, these foreign estrogens are adding to the increasing incidence of prostate cancer and benign prostatic hyperplasia.

It's almost impossible to avoid exposure to these chemicals since they are found everywhere. Dioxins, commonly used in pesticides and herbicides, are now found in our air and water. Ethanol (alcohol) and glycol ethers are used in glue, ink, antifreeze, sealants, and caulking compounds. Styrene is contained in the plastic used in food containers, carpets, and paper. Trichloroethylene is found in dry cleaning fluid, paint, and household cleaners, including drain cleaners.

Polychlorinated biphenyls (PCBs) were formerly used in hundreds of products, including plastics, carbonless copy paper, adhesives, and paints, and as flame retardants in children's pajamas and other items until they were banned in the 1970s. Another class of chemicals known as polybrominated diphenyl ethers (PBDEs) took their place and can be found in the foam of furniture cushions, plastics, automobiles, electronics, fabrics, and more.

Vinyl chloride, classified by the EPA as a human carcinogen, is used to make PVC and, in addition to being used in the products mentioned above, is found in plastic wraps for food, packaging materials, furniture and automobile upholstery, electronic devices, and many other common household and children's products. According to the EPA, exposure to high levels of this chemical has been shown to affect the central nervous system.

ELECTROMAGNETIC FIELDS

You are continually being exposed to electromagnetic field (EMF) radiation—another potentially dangerous element to the body—from x-rays, fluorescent lights, air travel, power lines, appliances, radar, television, electric blankets, cell phones, cordless phones, computers, Wi-Fi, Bluetooth headsets, microwaves, copiers, printers, hair dryers, and numerous other electrical devices. These low frequencies can pass through walls, floors, and your body and cause imbalances. The radiation destroys good bacteria in the body and creates damage from free radicals, both of which weaken the immune system and inflame the body.

CHAPTER SEVEN

PSYCHOLOGICAL AND SPIRITUAL STRESS

I n addition to all the chemical, dietary, and environmental factors that contribute to MS, we must also look at the role of psychological imbalances. Negative thinking, outdated beliefs, and fear-based emotions are major catalysts that suppress your immune system.

THE MIND-BODY CONNECTION

In the last several years we have heard a lot about the mind-body connection, which says that thoughts are things and that their energy directly impacts our bodies. We can no longer ignore this factor in our quest for health. Psychologist Shad Helmsetter says: "Leading behavioral researchers have told us that as much as 75 percent of everything we think is negative, counterproductive, and works against us. At the same time, medical researchers have said that as much as 75 percent of all illnesses are self-induced."[1]

Thoughts that emanate from your brain activate hormone secretions and stimulate nerve centers in the body. The resulting electrical impulses travel over the nerve fibers and trigger various bodily processes, including the glands and muscles, affecting your every motion and feeling every moment of every day. Simply stated, the thoughts that you think manifest your reality and the body that you walk around in.

YOUR THOUGHTS ARE IN
EVERY CELL OF YOUR BODY

Thoughts do not reside only in the brain. In reality, they are in every cell of your body. Each cell thinks and has its own memory. In his book *The Biology of Belief*, cell biologist Bruce Lipton talks about cellular intelligence. He writes about the important discoveries in this field by Candace Pert, an internationally recognized pharmacologist and neuroscientist: "*In Molecules of Emotion*, Pert revealed how her study of information-processing receptors on nerve cell membranes led her to discover that the same 'neural' receptors were present on most, if not all, of the body's cells. Her elegant experiments established that the 'mind' was not focused in the head, but was distributed via signal molecules to the whole body."[2]

The relatively new field of psychoneuroimmunology (PNI) studies the connection between the nervous system, the endocrine system, and the immune system and the effect that our mental states have on our immune response. For example, depression and stress have been shown to suppress the immune system. Therefore it follows that a chronic state of depression, in which the immune system is suppressed for a long period of time, can lead to disease.

The extensive research done in PNI and other fields makes it apparent that the body and mind are not separate. An illness may start in your mind and eventually affect your body, and vice versa. Every system and organ is interrelated. To categorize an illness as being either physiological or psychological is limiting. Once you understand the relationship between mind and body, you can take the necessary steps toward renewed health.

THE CONSCIOUS, SUBCONSCIOUS, AND UNCONSCIOUS MINDS

At a fundamental level, the mind consists of the conscious, subconscious, and unconscious. The conscious mind includes everything that we are aware of, and through it we communicate with the outside world. It's the place from which we exercise free will to discern and entertain thoughts of our choice.

The subconscious mind, which is just below our awareness, is like a huge computer bank that has stored in it every event that you've experienced in your lifetime. As the repository of all this information, it contains the habitual "programmed" physical and emotional responses we have learned from these past experiences. The subconscious mind does not know how to discern right from wrong, nor does it have a sense of humor. It is literal, and your best friend.

For instance, we've probably all had the experience of driving our car for several minutes on autopilot and all of a sudden realizing that we haven't been paying attention. Yet we managed to stop at the stop signs and turn at the right intersection to get home. What kept us from getting into a wreck or getting lost was our ability to access this previously learned information from the subconscious mind without having to consciously think about it.

The subconscious acts like a tape recorder that plays back the messages you've been programmed with since birth—that is, unless you change them. If as a child you were told that you'll never amount to anything, it's likely you've developed some limiting and self-defeating attitudes and beliefs. Unless recognized and discarded, negative and fear-based patterns will eventually play out in your body.

The unconscious mind contains all of the repressed emotions, urges, and memories that the conscious mind is unable to deal with. If you are harboring anger toward a parent for having emotionally or physically abused you, this emotion may be too painful for the conscious mind to acknowledge, and so it becomes buried in the unconscious. Even though we are consciously unaware of this material, it may still affect our behavior.

Most important to our discussion of health, your subconscious mind controls your central nervous system, which in turn controls every cell, tissue, and organ in your body. It regulates your involuntary bodily functions such as digestion, breathing, and circulation. With this understanding, you can work to access and change your subconscious beliefs so that they do not continue to sabotage your health. In Chapter 13 I will explain the different ways you can do this.

FEAR-BASED EMOTIONS

When examining our thoughts, we need to also look at our emotions and how the two work together. Thoughts feed emotions, and emotions feed thoughts. The two are inseparable, and if they are negatively based, they will create a vicious cycle that affects your health.

Most negative emotions are based on fear. If you examine emotions such as shame, anger, guilt, jealousy, rejection, and blame, you will likely find that fear is at the root of them. Unfortunately, throughout our lives we have often suppressed uncomfortable or painful emotions, though we still carry them around in the present as what many call "emotional baggage." The body has a cellular memory, and it retains this unresolved information. Over time, holding onto fear-based emotions, such as guilt or rage, will weaken your body. Therefore, it's important for you to feel these emotions and then let them go. You will find strategies for doing this in Chapter 13.

THE NATURE OF FEAR

Understanding the emotion of fear is especially important because it is a huge stressor that contributes to breaking down a body. Fear is the trickster, the culprit, the dragon, but it can also be one of your greatest teachers when you understand its origins.

What is fear? In some cases it's a natural response to a known danger or threat. However, in most cases in our lives fear takes the form of anxiety, which is an apprehension about what we think might happen in the future. Fear has been defined by some as *f*alse *e*vidence *a*ppearing *r*eal. In such cases, we may imagine the worst-case scenario, sometimes obsessively and in great detail, though we have absolutely no evidence of its reality.

There's a difference between survival fear and the fear you create in your mind based on false imagination. Feeling fear as you run across the street to escape an oncoming car is survival fear, or the fight-or-flight mechanism in action. It's instinctual and protective. On the other hand, fear of flying that originates from watching news stories about airplane crashes is a self-created fear and is destructive.

Fear dominates the lives of so many of us. Typically, our major fears are associated with death, money, relationships, illness, job security, and our purpose in life. Fear takes us out of our place of power, the now moment, since we're worrying about the future. The stress that results creates imbalances both psychologically and physiologically, sometimes causing panic attacks and often leading to disease. When you have MS, it's easy to be dominated by fear because something that you took for granted—your body functioning optimally—is now gone, and you fear what is coming next.

Many in the fields of spirituality and psychology tell us there are two primary emotions that we act from: love and fear. I believe this is true. In their book *Life Lessons*, psychiatrist Elisabeth Kübler-Ross and David Kessler say: "It's true that there are only two primary emotions, love and fear. But it's more accurate to say that there is only love or fear, for we cannot feel these two emotions together, at exactly the same time. . . . We have to make a decision to be in one place or the other. There is no neutrality in this. If you don't actively choose love, you will find yourself in a place of either fear or one of its component feelings."[3]

As contradictory as it may seem, choosing love means embracing our fear. An article on the Oprah.com website explains: "As long as you push away, deny or ignore fear, it will hold you captive and keep you emotionally frozen, unable to move forward. In that place, you become untrusting of love and spontaneity; you get angry or hide. But where fear contracts and closes the heart—resisting love—love expands and opens the heart, embracing fear."[4]

EVERY DISEASE HAS AN EMOTIONAL CORE

I believe that all diseases have an emotional component to them and that certain fear-based emotions correlate with the most common diseases of our time. For example, cancer has an emotional core related to feelings of repressed anger, guilt, or lack of self-love. MS is also related to repressed anger and low self-worth. Authors such as Carolyn Myss *(Anatomy of the Spirit)* and Louise Hay *(You Can Heal Your Life)* go into detail about how the core emotions we carry create various diseases.

In regard to those who have developed MS, Dr. Gabor Maté says that many MS patients share a characteristic childhood pattern in which their flight-or-fight response was blocked. In his book *When the Body Says No,* he explains that in the cases he has studied, these individuals "were exposed to acute and chronic stress by their childhood conditioning, and their ability to engage in the necessary flight-or-fight behaviour was impaired. The fundamental problem is not the external stress, such as the life events quoted in the studies, but an environmentally conditioned helplessness that permits neither of the normal responses of fight or flight. The resulting internal stress becomes repressed and therefore invisible. Eventually, having unmet needs or having to meet the needs of others is no longer experienced as stressful. It feels normal. One is disarmed."[5]

It is important to understand that the weight of our unresolved or repressed emotions will take its toll on the body unless we resolve these issues.

BELIEFS

Beliefs are ideas that we hold to be true. They are mostly stored in the subconscious, as I explained above, and are influenced by our experiences and environment. Beliefs are extremely powerful because they are the basis upon which you make choices and take action in the world. They affect how you think and feel. Most important, they can even change your DNA. Many scientists, including Bruce Lipton and Candace Pert, have done extensive research on how beliefs affect our biology.

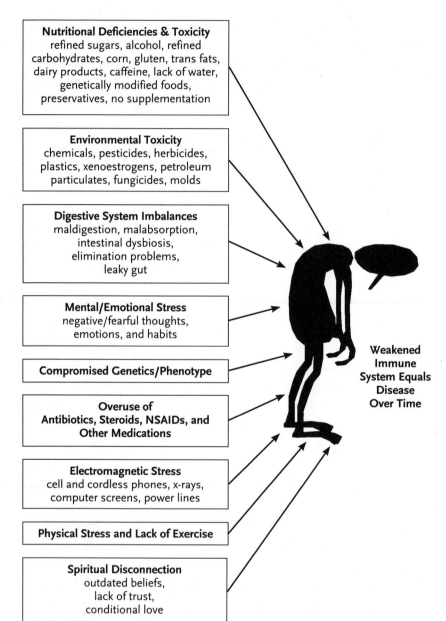

Nutritional Deficiencies & Toxicity
refined sugars, alcohol, refined
carbohydrates, corn, gluten, trans fats,
dairy products, caffeine, lack of water,
genetically modified foods,
preservatives, no supplementation

Environmental Toxicity
chemicals, pesticides, herbicides,
plastics, xenoestrogens, petroleum
particulates, fungicides, molds

Digestive System Imbalances
maldigestion, malabsorption,
intestinal dysbiosis,
elimination problems,
leaky gut

Mental/Emotional Stress
negative/fearful thoughts,
emotions, and habits

Compromised Genetics/Phenotype

**Overuse of
Antibiotics, Steroids, NSAIDs, and
Other Medications**

Electromagnetic Stress
cell and cordless phones, x-rays,
computer screens, power lines

Physical Stress and Lack of Exercise

Spiritual Disconnection
outdated beliefs,
lack of trust,
conditional love

Weakened
Immune
System Equals
Disease
Over Time

Figure 7.1: How Are You Stressed Out?

The bottom line: your beliefs impact your health. Holding on to limiting beliefs is damaging to your body and overall well-being. The good news is, beliefs are not laws written in stone. Like a worn-out tire, they can be changed when they become outdated and no longer get you where you want to go.

Unfortunately, most of your beliefs were ingrained in you at an early age when you did not have the conscious power of choice, and you have held on to them into your adult life. From your early childhood, you created a foundational picture of yourself. It didn't make any difference whether the pictures you created were true or not—you accepted what you heard and felt from your family, peers, and society as they defined who you were. Now it's time to change that definition.

SPIRITUAL DISCONNECTION

Your spiritual connection is essential to your health. It doesn't matter what religion or sect you belong to or what spiritual practices you do or do not do. All that matters is that you know you're connected to something greater than your body and mind. If you're an atheist, you can still believe in your own power to rise above physical or mental limitation and transform your life. Or you might have faith in a higher good that mankind can collectively aspire to. My experience has led me to believe that each of us has a "higher self," an all-knowing part of us that feels rightly and that we experience when we have hunches and follow our intuition.

It's important to understand that you are more than your body. Einstein showed that matter and energy are interchangeable, and physics tells us that energy never dies, but just changes form. Quantum physics has gone farther to show that matter is not really solid, that each atom is composed of a unique vibrating energy field, and that the combinations of these atoms make up everything in our "material" world, including our bodies.

I believe that each of us is a unique energy form called a soul and that we are part and parcel of a larger energy field that makes up the entirety of all that is. I call it God, Tao, or Universal Energy. It is this omnipresent, unseen force that becomes visible in such phenomenal events as the creation of a baby, the communication of cells with one another inside the body—and in the miraculous healings from "incurable" diseases.

What you believe and put your faith in will determine your outlook and quality of life. Your belief system affects your perceptions and the actions you take day in and day out and form the framework of how you operate. By identifying and discarding limiting beliefs, you allow yourself to open to unknown possibilities.

When I had MS, my hardest times were when I felt disconnected from God. I felt hopeless and full of anxiety, and I knew that if I remained hopeless, I would die. When we are spiritually disconnected we feel alone and isolated. This weakens us, leaving us open to imbalances, both physically, mentally, and emotionally. Depression, lack of self-worth, anxiety, hopelessness, and fear take greater hold when we lack faith in a power that is greater than ourselves to assist us with our healing.

THE NEXT STEP

The cumulative stress upon the body from nutritional, environmental, psychological, and spiritual causes can be devastating. See Figure 7.1 to recognize how they can stress you out. In Part Three I discuss ways to transform the negative patterns that have been set in motion in all of these areas so that you can start turning your health around.

PART THREE

YOU CAN HEAL YOURSELF: THE SOLUTIONS

CHAPTER EIGHT

THE CANDIDA CURE: A TWO-PRONGED STRATEGY

I n the United States, candidiasis is a silent epidemic that affects up to 80 million women, men, and children. In other words, one out of three people are afflicted with *Candida albicans* overgrowth.[1] Western medicine has persisted in ignoring this condition because its symptoms mimic so many other conditions and because it is, in large part, iatrogenic—that is, caused by physicians themselves through their overprescribing of antibiotics and other medications. Despite their denial, it is to be taken seriously because it is the main cause of MS and a host of other illnesses.

As I mentioned in Part One, I learned this through Dr. William Crook's book *The Yeast Connection*, which was a godsend when I went through my first health crisis at age nineteen. He was an expert on candida and his book describes it in detail. I've included his questionnaire in Part Four so you can score yourself and become aware of the symptoms you may be experiencing that correlate to candidiasis.

When beginning a program to eradicate this condition, the place to start is with your digestive system. In Chapter 5 you saw how maldigestion, malabsorption, and intestinal dysbiosis create the perfect breeding ground for *Candida albicans* over-growth and lead to leaky gut syndrome, which weakens the immune system and upsets the internal environment of the body. By way of leaky gut, *Candida albicans* overgrowth and its by-products filter into the bloodstream twenty-four hours a day and attack the most genetically vulnerable parts of your system. In the case of an MS patient, it is the central nervous system that is being attacked.

THE CANDIDA–IMMUNE SYSTEM CONNECTION

C. Orian Truss was another pioneering doctor who brought to our attention the severity of candidiasis and how our im-mune system can become paralyzed from fungal overgrowth. He states:

> The very existence of *Candida albicans* in the tissues on a chronic basis reveals an immune system at least par-tially "paralyzed" and "unresponsive" to its antigens— an immune system that is "tolerating" the continued presence in the tissues of the "foreign invader." Virtu-ally any organ seems susceptible to the effect of prod-ucts carried to it in the bloodstream, once released by the yeast after it has successfully invaded the tissues.[2]

The authors of *The Yeast Syndrome* explain the toll this takes on the body: "The passage of viable *Candida albicans* through the gastrointestinal (GI) mucosa into the host bloodstream is believed to be an important mechanism leading to systemic candidosis." They say that left untreated, *Candida albicans* "so severely debilitates the body that victims could become easy prey for far more serious diseases such as acquired immune deficiency syndrome, multiple sclerosis, rheumatoid arthritis, myasthenia gravis, colitis, regional ileitis, schizophrenia, and, possibly, death from candida septicemia."[3]

HOW TO IDENTIFY CANDIDA OVERGROWTH

The best way to know if you have *Candida albicans* overgrowth is to see a health-care practitioner who has experience treating this condition. By first completing Dr. Crook's questionnaire, you will start to see the connection between some of your MS symptoms and candidiasis. In my office, I examine my clients' responses to the questionnaire, take an extensive case history, and use various noninvasive testing techniques, including a quantum software program, to identify imbalances in their bodies.

If a client wishes, a blood test and/or stool test to detect *Candida albicans* overgrowth can also be done, but I usually discourage this. In my experience, I have found yeast and fungus to be evasive. They like to hide out in the organs and tissues, and therefore these tests give inconsistent results.

THE MYTH OF LAB TESTING

Due to many factors, lab tests are not always accurate. There are many unhealthy people whose blood work comes out negative because their conditions are subclinical. What this means is that even though they are symptomatic, their condition is undetectable on a blood test, and therefore they end up being misdiagnosed. Also, in general, the blood is the last system to show signs of imbalance, as the rest of the body will compensate in order to keep the blood levels normal, as I explained earlier.

For example, when it comes to survival, maintaining the proper blood pH of 7.35 is the body's priority. If the pH varies by even a few tenths of a percent, symptoms will appear, and if it varies by more than one-half of a pH unit, serious illness or death will occur. When the body compensates for a pH imbalance, other tissues and organs in the system may suffer. Your doctor may not even recognize these effects if he's just looking at blood test results.

Thus there are millions of unhealthy people running around with negative blood, urine, stool, and other lab results and not being treated. Many of my clients have had their doctors tell them, "There's nothing wrong" or "It's all in your head" because a set of tests came out negative. Blood, urine, and stool testing are only a few of the tools available for diagnosing a condition. If you're in this predicament, continue to search for the right health-care practitioner—someone who goes beyond lab tests to make a diagnosis.

Science, like any field, is on a learning curve and continuing to improve its technology to make more accurate diagnoses. However, the money and research that are necessary to develop better functional tests to diagnose candidiasis and other gut imbalances have been lacking because Western medicine has largely failed to recognize the true nature of these problems. Without accurate diagnostic testing, other methods must be used.

In the rare cases in which I do use blood and stool tests, even when the results come back negative I do not rule out treating the client for candidiasis in connection with MS, as I rely heavily on the other aspects of my evaluation. In fact, in all the years of my practice and seeing thousands of clients, I have let only a handful of people out of my office without starting them on a candida protocol. That's because using the protocol to first clear infection and inflammation from the client's body allows me to truly discover what other body systems are out of balance.

TREATMENT

The goal of treating candidiasis is to kill fungus and eradicate excess yeast. You never fully rid the body of yeast; you just get the levels back in balance. Achieving this balance requires a two-pronged strategy: taking an antifungal supplement to kill the fungus, and modifying your diet to starve the excess yeast. The treatment is simple, but takes diligence, discipline, and consistency on your part to achieve a successful outcome. Keep in mind that your body has an innate intelligence that allows it to heal itself. You simply need to give it the right environment.

ANTIFUNGALS

Taking an antifungal is critical to the success of your program. It can be either a pharmaceutical or herbal formula. Pharmaceuticals are more concentrated than herbal antifungals, and so with severe health conditions they can create faster changes. However, many of them are harsh on the liver.

The pharmaceutical antifungals include Nystatin, Diflucan (fluconazole), Nizoral (ketoconazole), Sporanox (itraconazole), and Lamisil (terbinafine). If you decide to use any of these, I recommend Nystatin, which is milder than the others, and/or Diflucan (for jump-starting only—see below). These two are the most effective in the program I have created.

Be aware that getting your doctor to prescribe a pharmaceutical antifungal can be challenging, especially if he or she isn't open to acknowledging the connection between yeast and

MS. Not to worry—herbal antifungals are just as effective and safer. Additionally, they act as antimicrobials and get rid of not only yeast, but parasites, bacteria, and viruses, all of which are involved in autoimmune diseases.

Pharmaceutical Antifungals

Nystatin: Nystatin is a concentrated extract of a soil-based organism that works by directly killing the yeast. Do not take Nystatin liquid; it contains sugar, which will feed the yeast.

As the authors of *The Yeast Syndrome* state: "Nystatin is virtually nontoxic and nonsensitizing. All age groups, including debilitated infants, accept the drug without demonstrating major side effects, even on prolonged administration. Most MS clients make the greatest progress after taking the medication for one to two years."[4]

Nystatin is not initially well absorbed into the bloodstream, but with prolonged use it does get into the blood and thus helps those with autoimmune diseases and cancer. The problem is that most doctors prescribe Nystatin for less than six weeks. Results are better if usage continues for six months or longer. When I was treating myself for MS, I took Nystatin for three years.

Diflucan (fluconazole): Diflucan is a synthetic antifungal drug that is effective against systemic candida overgrowth. It is ten times stronger than Nystatin, but also more toxic to the liver. If you use Diflucan or any other systemic antifungal (Nizoral, Sporanox, Lamisil) for more than a couple of weeks, have your doctor test and monitor your liver enzymes.

If you have symptoms of severe depression or anxiety, you can use Diflucan to jump-start the eradication of the fungus.

I suggest taking Diflucan for a limited time only, according to the dosage in the treatment protocol, and then switching to an herbal antifungal, such as Candida abX, or to Nystatin because they are safer. I also prefer Nystatin over Diflucan because it permeates the areas of the GI tract where yeast overgrowth usually originates, whereas Diflucan primarily targets the candida in the blood. To cure candidiasis, it is essential to tackle both the blood and the gut.

WARNING: If you are wheelchair bound or bedridden, Nystatin, Diflucan, and herbal antifungals are initially too strong for your body to handle. Since circulation is compromised and toxins do not move out of the body efficiently, probiotics are a safer choice.

Herbal Antifungals

Herbal antifungals are readily available and are safer than pharmaceuticals. You can find many of them at your local health food store, on Internet warehouse sites such as www.vitacost.com, www.annboroch.com, or at a health practitioner's office. In my practice, I have found the following to be the most effective for my clients:

- Candida abX (Quintessential Healing, Inc.)
- Candida Cleanse (Rainbow Light)
- pau d'arco (lapacho): liquid tincture, pills, or tea

All of these formulas have antifungal properties that target yeast overgrowth and also contain substances that are antibacterial, antiparasitical, and antiviral. Candida abX is well balanced and sharp in going after all microbial infections (see the Resources section on how to order this and other Quintessential Healing, Inc. products).

If you cannot find any of these antifungals in your local area, check the Resources section or look for yeast-eliminating products at your health food store that contain one or a mixture of some of the following ingredients:

- pau d'arco (lapacho)
- Oregon grape root
- garlic
- berberine sulfate
- undecylenic acid
- caprylic acid
- black walnut
- citrus seed extract
- oregano oil
- ginger
- gentian root
- marshmallow
- fennel

DIE-OFF REACTIONS

You need to be aware that starting a program of food elimination and taking an antifungal may create a Herxheimer reaction (also known as Jarisch-Herxheimer reaction) in which you experience die-off symptoms from killing the yeast. This detoxification process may make you feel worse before you feel better, and you may experience flu-like symptoms, headaches, body aches, abdominal distress, or a temporary worsening of your MS symptoms. To assist with this process, you need to make sure that all your elimination pathways—your liver, bowel, kidneys, lungs, and skin—are functioning optimally. In the next chapter, I discuss ways to do this. And in Part Four, you will find more detail on the nutritional supplements you will be taking to detoxify, support, and strengthen your body as you rid yourself of yeast overgrowth.

THE CANDIDA-CURE DIET

Eating the right foods is your second line of attack against yeast and fungal overgrowth. You will need to eliminate all sugars, dairy products, alcohol, gluten, and refined carbohydrates while you are taking an antifungal. In addition, you will need to eliminate all yeast and fermented products, even though they don't directly feed yeast. They often create an allergic or sensitivity response, so it is beneficial to eliminate them in the beginning of your treatment program.

Those who have a mild case of *Candida albicans* overgrowth can expect to feel better in six weeks to three months. People with autoimmune conditions, including MS, require from one to two years of taking an antifungal and following the diet to get the full benefits of the program. Remember, starving off the excess yeast requires both taking an antifungal and following the candida-cure diet for a long enough period of time. Trying to do one without the other will not produce positive results.

In Part Four, I put the components of the diet and the supplement program together so that you have a step-by-step guide to following the protocol.

HOW TO DEAL
WITH YOUR NEUROLOGIST

The best way to deal with your doctor is to educate yourself. Most doctors' knowledge is limited to what they have been taught in medical school, which is a drug-based approach to treating disease. If he or she doesn't agree with your choices, that's okay. Don't be intimidated. Remember that it's your body and you're in charge, so make decisions that feel right for you and that you feel peaceful about. If you make choices based on not wanting to disagree with your doctor or fear about what might happen if you don't follow his or her advice, you may end up prolonging your symptoms and hampering your recovery.

You may find that working solely with either Western or alternative medicine works best for you, or that you respond best to complementary medicine—a combination of Western and alternative approaches. No one way suits everyone. Each body is unique, and you need to listen to what yours is telling you.

Candida albicans overgrowth is real and is at the root of MS. It's so common that, as I said earlier, one out of three Americans have it in some form, from mild to severe.

WHAT IF I HAVE TO TAKE AN ANTIBIOTIC?

If your doctor prescribes an antibiotic and you choose to take it, ask for Diflucan or an antifungal of the same strength, three tablets total, to take after you finish the antibiotic. Take probiotics while on the antibiotic, but at a different time of the day. After your antibiotic course, take one Diflucan tablet every three days. Take the probiotics while you're taking the Diflucan, but at a different time, and continue the probiotics for one to two more months.

Doctors usually don't offer antifungals, but they need to be willing to give them to you if you ask. If your doctor won't give you three tablets, then just get one pill, as that is better than nothing. If you can't get Diflucan, just continue taking the antifungal you have been taking while on the program (e.g., Candida abX or Nystatin). If you are at the fourth month of the program or beyond and are in a month where you are taking only probiotics, add your herbal antifungal back in for a month, and take it at a different time of day than the probiotics.

If you are not ambulatory, but have started the antifungal and supplement protocol and are feeling stronger and eliminating daily, you should be able to handle the Diflucan or the herbal antifungal. However, if you are still weak and fragile or haven't started the program yet, use only the probiotics.

DON'T GIVE UP HOPE

Curing *Candida albicans* overgrowth requires both patience and discipline. If you find yourself feeling depressed in grocery stores and restaurants because they don't offer the food you can eat on your diet, shop at health food stores and online sites such as amazon.com or vitacost.com for the products listed in the back of this book. Not only will you find many wonderful choices, but you will also be eating more health-giving, nutritious foods.

Wherever you shop, be sure to read labels carefully, as even "health foods" sometimes contain sugar and ingredients you need to avoid while on the candida-cure diet.

It's best to approach getting rid of candida overgrowth as a lifestyle change rather than as a temporary fix. Once you feel better, you'll find that you are more sensitive to how food affects your body and mind, and ideally you won't want to go back to making poor food choices.

Persevere and the results will come. You will notice improvements in your health in as little as two to four weeks, and you will experience even greater changes after three to six months. Strict monitoring of your diet is essential. If you continue to eat sugar every day, even in small quantities, you will continue to feed the *Candida albicans* and your progress will be delayed. However, if you have a "bad day" and eat something that's not on your diet, don't beat yourself up. Just get back on your regimen and keep going.

STAYING WELL

As you restore your health, you will need to maintain it. To keep your body ecology balanced both during your candida treatment program and afterwards, you will need to reinoculate your gut by taking a dairy-free probiotic—a supplement that contains strains of "good bacteria," including acidophilus and bifidum. (See the instructions in Part Four.)

Curing candidiasis is a necessary first step in healing MS and it can take up to a minimum of two years or longer to bring yeast levels back into balance. Candida overgrowth can come back even more virulently if you go back to old habits of eating poorly. In cases of MS, you will need to take at least a reduced dose of an herbal antifungal compound for the rest of your life. You will also need to increase your dosage during stressful periods, such as when traveling and during holidays.

Even after you reach the end of the two-year period of clearing candida, you will need to live by a candida diet. Indulging in foods that contain sugar, dairy, yeast, gluten, and refined carbohydrates can easily reignite inflammation in the body. I highly advise avoiding alcohol permanently because of its neurotoxic effects on the central nervous system.

So, will you ever be able to cheat? The answer is yes, but only a little bit. There will be times of travel, holidays, parties, or just bad emotional days when you will want to eat what you want. Enjoy, and then get back on track. If you notice intolerances and reactions after eating any of these foods, such as a rapid pulse (90 to 180 beats per minute), fatigue, itching internally or externally, hives, gas, bloating, headaches, or a return of your MS symptoms, eliminate those foods entirely. This is a clear sign your body does not want them in your system.

NO SIDE EFFECTS

The good news about following the *Candida albicans* elimination protocol is that it can't harm you. It consists of only two major elements: cleaning up your diet and taking an antifungal supplement. This is a protocol that would benefit almost everyone, but especially those with autoimmune diseases. Many references are now available to help you educate yourself about this condition and about how to cook and eat properly. (See Part Four and Resources for more information.)

You have nothing to lose by choosing to treat candidiasis as a possible cause of your MS. You will have the information you need to monitor your progress and make sure the detox process is manageable. Certainly, making the choice to clean up your diet by eliminating sugar and refined and processed foods will make a difference in alleviating your symptoms.

CHAPTER NINE

INTERNAL DETOXIFICATION AND REMEDIES

YOUR BODY'S INTELLIGENCE

Your body is an amazing system that constantly works to keep you in homeostasis, a state of balance. It miraculously orchestrates communication of more than three hundred trillion cells. The body repairs and replaces cells day in and day out, year after year, decade after decade—including those in your skin, digestive tract, liver, and other organs.

Because of the body's inherent intelligence, my task is simply to assist my clients to make choices that will accelerate their natural healing mechanisms and to suggest ways they can strengthen their immune systems to overcome disease. Healing the body naturally means using nutritional therapy; hydrating your system; removing inflammation, infection, and toxins; and strengthening internal resistance.

Keeping your immune system strong is essential for health. The five main components of keeping your immune system healthy are quality sleep (six to eight hours), good nutrition, exercise, breathing, and meditation. Deep uninterrupted sleep repairs the body and mind. Nutritionally rich foods and supplements feed and repair your cells, tissues, and organs. Exercise not only keeps your body strong and agile, but alleviates distress and detoxifies your system. Breathing is by far the most important way to eliminate toxins because 75 percent of toxins are eliminated through the lungs compared to just 25 percent through urination, defecation, and perspiration combined. Focused deep breathing is thus a daily essential. Meditation is a practice that slows down the mind, relaxes you, and puts you into the "now" moment, your place of power.

In cases of autoimmune disease, a polluted internal environment has developed. Therefore, healing requires removing the accumulated wastes, free-radical damage, inflammatory agents, and antigens. To do this you need to incorporate detoxification methods that will clean up your gastrointestinal system, cleanse your liver and gallbladder, tonify your kidneys, and purify your blood and lymphatic system. You must also repair damaged tissues and organs by replenishing your body with nutrients. But diet alone is not enough. Repairing your nervous system and rebuilding your myelin sheath require an integrated regimen of both diet and supplementation that includes vitamins, minerals, and herbs.

TIME IS THE KEY

Having patience is of utmost importance during your healing process. Of all the body's systems, the central nervous system is one of the slowest to repair, so it's crucial that you set a realistic time frame for your treatment program. A person with MS who is ambulatory will usually heal faster than someone in a wheelchair, whose circulation is more compromised. Also, be aware that all people with MS don't experience exactly the same constellation of factors. This accounts for the differences in how fast symptoms abate and why one type of therapy or supplement works for one person and not another. It's important to individualize your treatment plan based on your unique body chemistry by working with your health-care practitioner or doctor.

DETOXIFICATION

Detoxification begins the process of removing inflammation, infection, and toxicity from your body. When you have MS, your body is delicate, so it's important to take it slow. The die-off from the candida and fungus can be intense for the first couple of weeks, with symptoms such as increased fatigue, headaches, cold-like or flu-like aches, and a worsening of your MS symptoms. These initial symptoms most often mean that you are on the right track, as toxins are releasing into the bloodstream.

The die-off symptoms usually pass within a couple of days to a week. However, if they are too intense, this indicates that the toxins aren't able to leave your body as fast as you're asking them to, so you will need to cut down on your dosage of the antifungal remedy and red clover tea. You may slowly increase the amounts again as you feel better. Stick with the program and work with a practitioner who knows how to deal with this process.

It's important to realize that there's a difference between an allergic reaction and a die-off reaction. With an allergic reaction, you will experience hives, swelling of the throat, or intense itching of the body. If you experience any of these symptoms, discontinue the antifungal, all supplements, and the tea. Wait three days to allow your body to calm down and then re-introduce the antifungal, each supplement, and the tea one at a time. Observe your body for two days before adding in another supplement or the tea. If you react again to a certain supplement or tea, cease taking that product altogether.

There's no need to rush your detoxification. Proceed at a pace that allows toxins to exit your body easily rather than ping-pong to other tissues and organs. If you are wheelchair bound or feel extremely weak, I suggest starting with the candida-cure diet and the slow-start program on page 355.

To help keep the toxins moving out of your system, it's also important to drink enough fluids in the form of water and herbal tea.

Improving Your Digestion

The first place to begin getting your body running smoothly is with your digestion. Start eating more uncooked, organic, and unprocessed food. Chew your food thoroughly and avoid eating in moments of extreme stress. If your digestion is severely imbalanced, you might need to steam or cook your vegetables in the beginning.

In addition, you might need to take digestive enzymes for the first couple of months to ensure that digestion is optimal and that undigested food particles aren't continuing to toxify your body. Enzymes assist with the proper breakdown of food and get rid of symptoms of indigestion, heartburn, gas, and bloating.

If you have trouble digesting animal protein (burping and heartburn), buy an enzyme that contains pepsin and hydrochloric acid (HCl). If you have blood-sugar imbalances (low or high), use a pancreatic enzyme that contains pancreatin, lipase, protease, and amylase. If you're vegetarian or have mild digestive complaints, use a plant-based digestive enzyme. Good brands of enzymes are Super Digestaway (Solaray), Enzy-Gest (Priority One), and Digest Gold (plant-based, Enzymedica).

Cleansing Your Colon

Second in importance is making sure your bowels move daily. Your colon walls have been affected by years of stress, poor diet, and internal and external pollutants. It's important to remove this cumulative buildup. One bowel movement a day is mandatory, and two to three are ideal.

The keys to keeping your bowels moving daily are drinking enough water (one-half of your body weight in ounces per day), taking the time to move your bowels when you have the urge, exercising regularly, and making sure to get enough fiber in your diet.

Fiber is beneficial for sweeping the linings of your colon and keeping elimination optimal. You can get additional fiber by using a supplement with citrus pectins, flaxseed, chia seed, or rice bran. Gentle Fibers (Jarrow) and FiberSMART (ReNew Life) are good sources and may be used daily for bowel regularity. Take one level tablespoon in ten ounces of water. After the first week, increase the dosage to two tablespoons if necessary. All of these are available in health food stores or online at www.vitacost.com. Psyllium is another fiber source that works well for some people. However, because psyllium expands to forty times its volume, it can cause more bloating and gas. I usually recommend psyllium for cases of diarrhea and not for constipation.

Even if you are consuming adequate amounts of fiber in fruits and vegetables and are eliminating daily, I recommend taking added fiber in the form of ground flaxseed. It not only assists you to eliminate each day, but also removes toxins such as mucus, yeast, and other by-products that have built up on your colon walls. Fiber may be used indefinitely.

If fiber is not doing the trick and you are still constipated, you need to ensure a daily bowel movement some other way.

Otherwise your die-off symptoms from taking an antifungal are likely to intensify. Mild laxatives you can try are Magnesium Citrate (Life Extension) or Triphala (Planetary Herbals or Himalaya), which are good formulas that can be used long term if needed. Start by taking one pill (or one teaspoon if powder) after dinner and increase your dose daily by one pill until you achieve daily bowel movements. Triphala can be spread out throughout the day; magnesium is best taken after dinner. Be sure not to take so much that you have loose stools or diarrhea. The goal is to have full, normal, formed stools on a daily basis. Adjust the dose until it is right for you.

For moderate and severe cases of constipation, try Aloe Lite or Aloe 225 (BioDesign), or Dr. Christopher's Quick Colon Formula Part I. Take one pill after dinner and increase your dose daily by one pill until you achieve daily bowel movements. Aloe Lite and Aloe 225 may be used long term. Dr. Christopher's may be used for up to six months.

Stubborn and long-term cases of constipation can also benefit from high colonic irrigation treatments. Usually a series of three treatments is enough to accelerate the detoxification process. These treatments can restore bowel motility so that you have movements daily. Colonics are not advisable if you have ulcers, Crohn's disease, ulcerative colitis, or diverticulitis.

Deep Breathing and Releasing Toxins through the Skin

Because 75 percent of the toxins you eliminate will leave your body through your lungs, it's important to do deep breathing exercises several times a day. Focus on your belly and let it expand as you inhale to a count of seven; hold the breath for a count of seven; and then exhale slowly, contracting your belly, to a count of seven. Do this for two minutes four times a day.

Sweating out toxins is also helpful. For some people with

MS, an infrared sauna is the only kind of sauna the body can tolerate; those who are more progressed should avoid them. Avoid regular dry or steam saunas because they heat up the body's core and will make your symptoms worse.

Cleansing Your Gallbladder and Liver

While you are detoxifying, your liver will need extra attention to make sure that it is able to properly filter the toxins you are releasing. Therapeutic cleansing herbs and therapies will help your overtaxed liver to recover so it can do an efficient job of neutralizing internal and external poisons and also ensure that these toxins don't recirculate in your system.

The gallbladder works closely with the liver and also needs supplementation. During the first month of your program take a gallbladder formula, such as Gallbladder abX (Quintessential Healing, Inc.), to stimulate bile secretion, eliminate toxins, and improve fat digestion. For the second and third months of the program, take a liver formula, such as Liver abX (Quintessential Healing, Inc.), to help with liver detoxification. If you are not able to obtain the products listed above, find ones that contain some of the following: milk thistle seed, dandelion root, N-acetylcysteine, minerals, turmeric, B vitamins, artichoke leaf, beet root, ginger, choline, taurine.

Tonifying Your Kidneys and Cleansing Your Bloodstream

The next vital step is to make sure the blood is cleansed by ridding it of toxins, including heavy metals and mycotoxins from yeast/fungus. Drinking two to four cups of red clover tea daily will assist with this and also with cleansing the kidneys and bladder. Many people with MS suffer from urinary incontinence or urgency, so in the beginning you may be making even more trips to the bathroom, but eventually you'll see the benefits. If overactivity and urgency is still a problem, reduce the amount of red clover tea to one-half cup daily. If overactivity persists, stop drinking it altogether. (Do not drink red clover tea if you have ulcers, acid reflux, or grass allergies, or if you are on blood-thinning medication.)

If you experience recurring urinary tract infections, try U.T. Vibrance (Vibrant Health) or a product with cranberry, uva ursi, marshmallow, and/or slippery elm. Another helpful remedy is D-mannose, a naturally occurring simple sugar that knocks out *Escheria coli* (E. coli) bacteria that attach to the bladder walls. D-mannose coats E. coli so it can no longer stick to the tissues. It doesn't disrupt blood-sugar levels or feed candida and can be taken long term.

Stimulating Your Lymphatic System

Last but not least is keeping your lymph moving optimally. The lymphatic system's main job is to move waste out of the body's tissues. Unlike the heart, it does not have a pumping mechanism and relies on your body's gravity and movement to push the lymph fluid through its vessels all the way to the heart area, where the collecting ducts dump the waste into the bloodstream.

Because it relies on the movement of your body, the best ways to cleanse the lymphatic system are by exercising regularly, doing daily deep-breathing exercises, getting massages once a month, and skin brushing.

Dry skin brushing is a simple yet effective way to stimulate the lymph system. Buy a natural fiber, long-handled brush from your local health food store. Before getting into the shower each morning, brush your skin with short, gentle upward strokes, starting from the bottom of your feet and moving up. Always brush toward your heart. Your lymph fluid is right under your skin, so you don't need to brush hard. Brush up your legs, your torso, and back, and then over your shoulders down to the heart (center of your chest). Brush your fingers and up your arms. Do not brush your face, as the bristles can scratch facial skin. You may be able to handle soft strokes from the neck down toward your heart. Brush for a total of three to five minutes. You will start to feel your circulation increasing, and you may feel a tingling sensation. Skin brushing also helps your skin to start new cell growth. After your shower or bath, massage your body with coconut, almond, or jojoba oil while your skin is still moist.

Finally, exercise if you can. This will stimulate the lymphatic system to detox. Brisk walking, swimming, isometric exercises, qigong, or yoga is sufficient.

IMPROVING YOUR CIRCULATION

Optimal circulation is essential for ridding your central nervous system of waste and moving nutrients into your organs and tissues for repair. One of the most effective ways to improve your circulation is by bringing more oxygen into your body, which can be achieved by exercising and breathing exercises. Skin brushing also increases circulation.

Ginger, gingko biloba, niacin, and hawthorn berry will also help improve your circulation. In Part Four I will explain how to work these into your supplement regime. Oxygen therapy, ionic footbaths, and enzyme therapy are also adjunctive ways to support circulation and accelerate the removal of inflammation from the body.

NOTE: Do not take gingko biloba if you are on blood-thinning medication. If you will be having surgery, stop taking gingko two weeks before so your blood will clot properly.

OXYGEN THERAPY

Oxygen is also beneficial because it creates an environment that's hostile to pathogenic microbes and helps regenerate nerve cells. Hyperbaric oxygen treatment (HBOT) is one method for alleviating oxygen deficiency, thereby improving circulation, neutralizing toxins, renewing sleeping (dormant) neurons, stimulating neural stem cells, encouraging new blood vessel growth into damaged tissues, and reducing brain swelling. There are two types of HBOT—mild HBOT, which uses lower atmospheric pressure, and higher pressure HBOT. Finding a place that offers mild HBOT will be easier and less expensive. Usually a series of five to ten sessions is needed in order to see a benefit.

IONIC FOOTBATHS

The rate at which bodies are able to eliminate toxins can be slow, especially if you are not ambulatory. To assist with the process, ionic footbaths are extremely beneficial. I feel they are a necessity to keep up with the overload of heavy metals, chemicals, and pollutants we are taking in from food, air, and water.

Ionic footbaths create negative and positive ions, which assist with removing heavy metals and toxins, increasing blood circulation, killing bacteria and fungus, increasing oxygen in the body, relieving pain, improving sleep, and balancing the immune system. Footbaths are gentle and noninvasive. You simply put your feet into a small tub of warm water that has an ionic device situated between your feet. Depending on the manufacturer of the unit, each session lasts from fifteen to thirty minutes. I recommend doing only one session a week. Those in your family who are healthy and want to achieve the benefits of doing a footbath can do it once every ten days.

You can look for a practitioner who offers this treatment or purchase a unit. The brand I sell is the Ionic S.P.A., which will give you 250 to 300 footbaths (see Resources).

RELIEVING SPASTICITY, PAIN, DEPRESSION, AND ANXIETY

Cannabis (marijuana) is one of the most therapeutic herbs for these issues, but it is not available to the public. When medical marijuana can be obtained, it may be used to decrease spasticity and tremors, alleviate pain, eliminate insomnia, and relieve anxiety and depression. The best way to use this herb is as a tea, not by smoking it, which can damage cells. Another tea that may help with spasticity is a honey-rosemary tea cocktail. In Part Four I include instructions for preparing both of these remedies, and also list supplements that are specifically designed to relieve spasticity, pain, depression, and anxiety.

ENZYME THERAPY

Enzymatic therapy accelerates the body's healing and is critical for those with MS, especially during an exacerbation or a bout of optic neuritis, because it can eliminate the need for steroids.

While digestive enzymes are designed to digest food and improve assimilation, systemic (or metabolic) enzymes help the body better perform certain metabolic processes. These include decreasing inflammation, decomposing toxins, improving circulation, purifying the blood, fighting viruses, speeding up tissue repair, stimulating immunity, removing scar tissue and plaque in the veins and arteries, and strengthening and restoring the body's general resistance. Systemic enzymes are formulated so that they are not destroyed by stomach acid and need to be taken on an empty stomach, whereas digestive enzymes must be taken with food.

Another function of enzyme therapy is to destroy circulating immune complexes, which occur at higher levels in people with MS. The immune system recognizes fungi, bacteria, and viruses as enemies (antigens) and produces antibodies. When the antibodies couple with the antigens they form immune complexes that circulate in the bloodstream and/or fix themselves to tissues in the body, where they do damage. In those with MS, they can attack the myelin sheath, and therefore enzyme therapy may be beneficial.

Trevinol Professional is the best enzyme to use. It contains serrapeptase, bromelain, nattokinase, protease, papain, lactobacillus sporogenes (585 million CFU), quercetin, coenzyme Q10, alpha-lipoic acid, magnesium, and vegetable cellulose. (See Part Four, Second Month, for dosing information.) The improvements that you're looking for with this therapy are more energy; decreased spasticity, pain, and inflammation; increased range of motion and mobility; quicker subsiding of exacerbations; and an overall lightness within the body.

NOTE: Enzymes thin the blood and slow coagulation, so enzyme therapy is not recommended for pregnant women or those with ulcers, gastritis, hemophilia, or extremely low blood pressure, or for those on blood-thinning medication or aspirin.

REBUILDING YOUR MYELIN SHEATH

While you're treating candidiasis, it's also important to focus on rebuilding your myelin sheath. According to neurologist David Perlmutter, "Creating the most advantageous environment for repair and regeneration of myelin requires an adequate supply of EFAs [essential fatty acids]. About 75 percent of myelin is composed of fat, with a substantial amount coming from the essential fatty acids."[1]

Lipids, which include fats, form part of the sheath of the brain and are also found in nerve and muscle cells. Therefore, omega-3 and omega-6 essential fatty acids need to be taken daily because they're the building blocks of brain and nerve tissue. You can get them from foods such as raw nuts and seeds, cold-water fish (sardines, mackerel, salmon—preferably wild, not farmed), dark-green leafy vegetables, and legumes. However, in order to reach therapeutic levels you also need to take EFAs in liquid supplement form. I recommend high-quality products such as High Concentrate EPA-DHA Liquid (Metagenics), Very Finest Fish Oil (Carlson), or Ultimate Omega Liquid (Nordic Naturals). The therapeutic dosage is two teaspoons to one tablespoon daily.

Another essential part of the myelin sheath, as well as the cell membranes, is EAP (ethanol-amino-phosphoric acid). Chelated calcium, magnesium, and potassium EAP are found in the German mineral formulation called Mynax (Koehler USA). EAP assists in repairing myelin and with the proper firing of neurons, and is critical for balancing the central nervous system, which may result in the alleviation of MS symptoms such as muscle spasms, tremors, fatigue, moodiness, and headaches.

Note: Do not take fish oil if you are on blood-thinning medication. If you will be having surgery, stop taking the fish oil two weeks before so your blood will clot properly.

NUTRIENTS FOR CENTRAL NERVOUS SYSTEM REPAIR

Crucial supplements for restoring central nervous system function are vitamins C and E. Vitamin C is an antioxidant that protects the brain and spinal cord from free-radical damage and strengthens the immune system. Vitamin E, another antioxidant, improves oxygen utilization, protects cell membranes from free-radical attack, and also enhances the immune system.

Dosages for those with MS need to be higher than for the average person. Therapeutic levels of vitamin C range between 3,000 to 6,000 milligrams (3 to 6 grams) daily. Doses of vitamin E are between 800 and 1,200 IU (international units) daily for those who are ambulatory, and 2,000 IU for those who are bedridden or wheelchair bound. Use a full-spectrum E with all tocopherols and tocotrienols

The following supplements are also beneficial for healing the central nervous system: acetyl-L-carnitine, grape seed extract, all the B vitamins (particularly B12), N-acetylcysteine, phosphatidylcholine, phosphatidylserine, vitamin D3, CoQ10, alpha lipoic acid, turmeric, resveratrol, broccoli seed extract, black pepper extract, pterostilbene, green tea leaf extract, pine bark extract, and gingko biloba.

Combination formulas that include some of the items above are Brain Vitale Powder (Designs for Health), Nrf2 Activator (Xymogen), Acai Resveratrol Ultimate ORAC Antioxidant Extreme (HealthForce Nutritionals), NeuroActives Brain Sustain (Xymogen), and NeuroTone (Douglas Labs). Taking one of these will reduce the quantity of pills you need to swallow. In Part Four I will give more detailed guidance about the supplements you will be taking.

NOTE: Do not take vitamin E or gingko biloba if you are on blood-thinning medication. If you will be having surgery, stop taking vitamin E and gingko two weeks before so your blood will clot properly. If you begin to noticeably bruise, reduce your dose of vitamin E.

TREATING VIRUSES, BACTERIA, AND PARASITES

The solution to ridding your body of microbial infections is to eliminate their food supply. Viruses, bacteria, and parasites, as well as yeast/fungus, all thrive on sugar. Eliminating sugar from your diet is essential to stop infection in your body. By following the candida-cure diet and antifungal protocol, you'll kill off more than just candida and fungus—you'll also be treating viruses, parasites, and bacteria. Viruses will become dormant, unhealthy bacteria and parasites will be eliminated, and yeast will be put back into a balanced ratio.

However, some bacterial infections require additional treatment. If you test positive for *Chlamydia pneumoniae*, a bacterial infection, the best course of action is to take an antibiotic called doxycycline. Ask your doctor to prescribe it at 100 milligrams twice a day for fourteen to twenty-one days. To keep yeast in check while you're taking it, be sure to take an antifungal, such as Nystatin or Candida abX, or probiotics that contain multistrains of acidophilus and bifidus.

If you test positive for Lyme disease (caused by a bacteria carried by ticks), effective remedies are cat's claw, colloidal silver (www.silver100.com), teasel, and/or pau d'arco (lapacho). Pau d'arco is a powerful antimicrobial herb and is effective in ridding the body of viruses, bacteria, yeast/fungus, and parasites. Antibiotic therapy is usually recommended for treating this disease, so if you decide to use this method, make sure to take an antifungal while you're on the antibiotics.

Lyme disease is challenging to diagnose and can be mistaken for MS. The biggest difference between the two is that extreme joint pain presents with Lyme disease. The best lab for diagnosing Lyme disease is IGeneX (www.igenex.com). I also suggest finding a physician who specializes in its treatment instead of trying to deal with this condition on your own.

AMALGAM REMOVAL
AND CHELATION THERAPY

The best indicator of high mercury levels in the body is a urine test. Second best is a hair analysis. If you decide to have your silver-mercury fillings removed, work with a dentist who has experience doing this procedure. Be sure that he or she follows proper protocol by using a dental dam to prevent particles of mercury from going under your tongue, and by having you wear a mask so mercury vapors don't go up your nose during drilling.

When replacing your fillings, one option is to work with a dentist who tests for materials that are compatible with your body. However, this can get quite expensive, so it's up to you. I have found that composite fillings, ones that match the color of your teeth and are made of plastic, are the easiest and next-best choice.

Even if you use a mask and a dental dam, mercury vapors will still leach into the body. Therefore it is essential to chelate, or pull out, the metal residues afterwards. Red clover tea is one of the best chelators. It will pull the mercury residue from your organs and tissues and clean up your blood, kidneys, and liver. Drink one quart of red clover tea daily during and after the procedure and for three months after your last fillings have been removed. (Do not drink red clover tea if you have ulcers, acid reflux, or grass allergies, or if you are on blood-thinning medication.)

Another chelating agent is cilantro, which mobilizes mercury and other heavy metals. You can take it in liquid tincture form or add it fresh to vegetable juice. When you take cilantro, you also need to take a type of algae called chlorella to transport the metals out of your body. I recommend using both together for one month after amalgam removal.

After your three months of drinking red clover tea, I highly recommend taking Natural Cellular Defense by Waiora. It contains zeolite, a volcanic mineral that chelates heavy metals without pulling out the good minerals, such as calcium, magnesium, potassium, etc. Work up slowly to ten drops three times a day in eight ounces of water, with or without food. You need only buy one three-pack, which will last for six to eight weeks. If you take Natural Cellular Defense, do not drink red clover tea or take the liquid cilantro and chlorella, as this would be too much chelation at once.

If you are considering removing your amalgam fillings, wait at least six months to one year after starting the candida-cure diet and detox program so that a substantial portion of the infection and inflammation are cleared out of your system. The goal is to help the body be in a stronger position to handle the possible detoxifying effects of having the metals removed. Avoid removing your fillings if you are not ambulatory or are very weak, because the toxic mercury vapors will put too much stress on your body.

Even if you don't have amalgam fillings, heavy metals have accumulated in your body from the air you breathe and the food and water you take in, so chelation at some point would be beneficial. In addition to what is listed above, ionic footbaths are an important adjunct in removing heavy metals.

BALANCING BLOOD SUGAR
AND ADRENAL FUNCTION

In my years of practice, I have found that the most common imbalances in my clients are in their blood-sugar levels and in their adrenal function, which are givens in those with autoimmune disease. Low blood sugar is called hypoglycemia. Symptoms associated with it are feeling irritable, light headed, and/or shaky if meals are missed; having cravings for sweets during the day; being forgetful; having blurry vision; and experiencing highs and lows of energy throughout the day (usually low energy in the afternoon). High blood sugar, also known as diabetes or insulin resistance, exhibits as fatigue after meals, a craving for sweets after meals, and an ability to skip meals and still function.

I feel it is essential to balance blood-sugar levels in those with MS at the beginning of their program. To do so equates to better digestion, consistent energy, improved balance/gait, and clearer focus throughout the day. Following the candida-cure diet will bring blood-sugar levels into balance. In addition, I suggest using an herbal-vitamin supplement called Gluco abX (Quintessential Healing, Inc.) for the first couple of months to help eliminate hypoglycemia, improve energy, and reduce sugar and carbohydrate cravings, thereby helping you stick to the candida-cure diet.

The adrenals are triangle-shaped glands that sit atop your kidneys. They help you to manage stress and to survive by kicking into high gear and secreting hormones when you are in fight-or-flight mode. Unmanaged stress is the number-one reason the adrenals become fatigued. Next in line are caffeine and sugar consumption. Symptoms that exhibit with adrenal imbalance are fatigue, dizziness, low blood pressure, anxiousness, craving for salt, inability to focus, insomnia, and even panic attacks. I recommend taking Adrenal abX (Quintessential Healing, Inc.) during the second and third months of the program to help balance and replenish the adrenal glands and endocrine system, and also to restore energy levels. After the third month, adaptogenic herbs such as holy basil, ashwagandha, rhodiola, and eleuthero root are good to take to secure healthy adrenal function.

Blood sugar and adrenal function have a symbiotic relationship. The more stressed out you are, the more your adrenal glands will secrete adrenaline and cortisol. These inflame the body and elevate glucose, which can bring on hypoglycemia. The more your diet is filled with caffeine, sugar, alcohol, and junk food, the more imbalanced blood sugar becomes, stressing the body and depleting the adrenals. Eventually you wind up craving and eating more sweets and carbohydrates and taking stimulants to stay even or keep going. This vicious cycle feeds candida because yeast don't care if the elevated glucose is coming from eating a brownie or from feeling stressed about trying to make your mortgage payment.

SLEEP

Getting six to eight hours of quality sleep each night is necessary to repair and replicate healthy cells. It is the first and foremost factor in repairing an immune system. Ideally, you want to go to bed by 10 p.m. because from 10 p.m. to 2 a.m.

your body makes physiological repairs. From 2 a.m. to 6 a.m. psychological repair takes place. If you can't go to bed by 10 p.m., at least try to lie down so that your body is in rest position until you do go to sleep.

If you have trouble falling asleep or staying asleep, drink a cup of organic chamomile tea (steeped for twenty minutes) one hour before bed, or use natural products such as Tranquil Sleep (Natural Factors), 5 HTP (Jarrow), Benesom (Metagenics), Melatonin, 1 mg (Life Extension, Jarrow), or a homeopathic formula such as Calming (Heel/BHI). It is also beneficial to have some protein at dinner to help stabilize blood sugar and prevent it from dipping too low. Hypoglycemia is often the reason that people wake up between the hours of 1 and 3 a.m.

Doing breathing exercises or playing hypnosis or subliminal CDs that assist with insomnia or healing can also help you fall asleep. Make sure your room is as dark as possible so that the pineal gland can produce optimal levels of melatonin, a powerful antioxidant that aids sleeping.

CHAPTER TEN

NUTRITION: REGENERATING YOUR TOXIC AND DEPLETED BODY

A HEALTHY DIET

When I give workshops, people frequently ask, "Since so many foods cause cancer, what should I eat and drink?" It's true that your body has to adapt more than ever before because of the pollutant overload in our foods and environment, but you don't need to walk around in fear—the body can handle more than you think. Yet there is a tipping point. Your body will start to shut down if you compound the problem by abusing it with poor dietary choices, living in a polluted environment, putting your energy into negative thoughts and emotions, and continually operating at high stress levels.

So what is a healthy diet? It's one that consists of 60 percent organic vegetables; 20 percent meat and fish that are antibiotic- and hormone-free (meat from grass-fed animals); 15 percent gluten-free whole grains; and 5 percent organic fruits, nuts, seeds, beans/legumes (avoid for first three months of the program), and unrefined oils. By adopting a diet of wholesome, unprocessed food and pure water, you can begin to starve out the MS disease process and help the healthy cells and tissues of your organs to replicate.

It's essential for you to know which foods are beneficial and which ones to avoid. Fruits, vegetables, and plant foods are abundant in phytochemicals, which help prevent cancer and reverse disease. The most important vegetables to consume daily are dark-green leafy vegetables (spinach, watercress, collard greens, mustard greens, poke greens, turnip greens, dandelion greens, arugula, baby greens, bok choy, kale, etc.) and sprouts. They are filled with vitamins and minerals, especially B_6 and magnesium, that are required for your body's many metabolic processes. Cruciferous vegetables, such as broccoli, brussels sprouts, and cauliflower, contain natural compounds that assist with healthy liver function. Raw nuts and seeds contain essential fatty acids needed by the membrane around each cell.

The more we discover about the beneficial compounds in our whole foods, the clearer it becomes that eating a healthy diet is essential. By doing so, you stop the progression of disease and reduce the amount of supplementation you need to maintain your health.

ORGANIC FOOD

The synthetic pesticides, fungicides, and herbicides used on conventionally grown foods, including genetically modified foods, are carcinogenic. As discussed in Chapter 6, even though science hasn't fully disclosed all the negative effects that GMO foods have on our bodies, they should be avoided because of the toxic chemicals used to produce them.

You can avoid chemicals and get the best-quality nutrients by supporting certified organic farmers and eating organic fruits, vegetables, and meats. These foods are more expensive, but you and your health are worth the investment. Quality outweighs convenience when it comes to healing your body. Be sure to wash all your fruits and vegetables with a little soap and water or a natural fruit-and-vegetable wash, which you can find in the health food store.

VEGETARIAN DIET

Vegetarians make a number of valid points about the negative aspects of eating meat. It's true, unfortunately, that animals are treated inhumanely and that the use of hormones and antibiotics is widespread. Yet I find that eating some animal protein each week is the easiest way to keep your body in balance. It's also necessary since 50 percent of the body's nonwater mass is made up of protein.

For MS patients, it is especially important to make sure your body is sustaining muscle mass; otherwise you will become weak and frail. Eating small servings of lean animal protein, such as chicken, turkey, and fish, helps to avoid this problem. On the other hand, saturated fat in red meat can increase inflammation in your body, particularly when cooked past medium-rare and eaten with starches and grains. Because MS is an inflammatory condition, it's therefore better to avoid it or to consume it in small amounts.

Vegetarianism is a personal choice that only you can make. If you decide to become a vegetarian, or already are one, educate yourself. Most of my vegetarian clients are unhealthy because they're not compensating for nutrients they are lacking that can only be found in meat, such as certain amino acids and B vitamins. Also, I find that their diets often contain excessive amounts of refined carbohydrates and sugar, which deplete vitamins and minerals and feed candida, leading to degeneration in the body.

WHOLE GRAINS

Whole grains are complex carbohydrates that have not been bleached or stripped of their fiber. They include amaranth, barley, brown rice, wild rice, buckwheat, corn, kamut, millet, quinoa, oats, rye, spelt, teff, triticale, and whole wheat.

Grains contain important B vitamins that keep your central nervous system in balance. They also have fiber, which is important for helping with daily bowel elimination and keeping the colon lining healthy. The problem is that most of us eat too much from this food group, when we only need 25 to 50 grams of carbohydrates a day.

I do not recommend corn because it has a high sugar content and most of it is genetically modified, or gluten grains—barley, kamut, oats (unless gluten-free), rye, spelt, triticale, and wheat—because they create an inflammatory response in the body, especially in people with autoimmune conditions.

GOOD FATS

There are major differences between good fats and bad fats (trans fats). The good fats help to regulate hormones, blood pressure, heart rate, and nerve transmission, as well as reduce inflammation and pain. Your body needs good fats such as omega-3s, omega-6s, and omega-9s because it uses them to coat every cell membrane, and the integrity of the membranes ensures the proper nutrition of your cells. Your body does not manufacture the omega-3 and omega-6 essential fatty acids on its own and only manufactures a limited amount of omega-9s, so you must include them in your daily diet.

Foods high in omega-3 essential fatty acids include deep-sea fish, dark leafy greens, coconut, flax, fish oil, hempseed oil, krill oil, olive oil, raw nuts and seeds, and avocados. Organic butter contains small amounts of omega-3s as well as vitamins A and D (use unsalted). To repair your myelin sheath and reduce inflammation, it's essential to eat foods high in omega-3s and to also take them in supplements, as you won't obtain enough through your diet.

Omega 6 essential fatty acids are found in eggs, grass-fed meat, raw nuts and seeds, and safflower, sunflower, and hemp oils. Here, too, you need additional supplementation. The best source of omega-9 fatty acids is olive oil, but they can also be found in almonds, avocados, and sesame oil.

Saturated fats from foods such as eggs, coconut meat and oil, butter, ghee (clarified butter), raw goat cheese (eat only after first three months of your program), and grass-fed red meat are beneficial in small quantities. These foods contain important vitamins and minerals, but you should eat them in moderation because large quantities can make the body more inflamed.

Don't be fooled by the claims made about all the low-fat foods on the market and think they are good for you. They often contain high concentrations of chemicals and refined sugars.

ANIMAL PROTEIN

During the digestive process, animal protein breaks down into amino acids, which your body needs for regenerating and repairing cells, tissues, and organs. Most people with MS do best having small amounts of animal protein daily. This also helps to keep blood-sugar levels balanced. Consuming animal protein fewer than three times a week will create deficiencies in your body. If you are a vegetarian, become educated about how to balance proteins and carbohydrates, and about which supplements to take to compensate for the protein deficit.

Eat lean animal protein such as chicken, turkey, and fish in small amounts (2–4 ounces a day or at least three times a week). Eggs are also a good source of protein and are best prepared poached, soft-boiled, sunny-side up, or hard-boiled. As much as possible, make sure your meat and eggs are from free-range animals who are not given hormones and who are either grass-fed or whose feed is vegetarian and antibiotic- and GMO-free. Free-range chickens are not confined in small cages and may have a little more room to move around than chickens that are raised on factory farms. However, their conditions are not necessarily humane or sanitary and they are often kept in crowded sheds or lots. Ideally, the best meat to eat is from animals who are pasture raised, where they are truly free to roam outdoors. Finding this type of meat, though, can be a challenge, so you will have to do the best you can given your resources.

As mentioned above, it's usually best to avoid red meat because of the inflammation factor, but some body types do well on small amounts. If you do eat it, choose meat from grass-fed animals, such as bison, and eat it only once a week. Listen to your body to feel if you're craving meat. When preparing red meat, cook it rare to medium-rare, as this leaves some active enzymes to help you digest it, and do not eat it with starchy vegetables or grains, as this will make your body acidic. If you are still not digesting the meat well, use a protein digestive enzyme that contains HCl and pepsin.

Avoid tuna of any kind and all shellfish because of their high mercury levels. All fish contain some heavy metals, yet I feel that their benefit as a good source of omega-3 fatty acids outweighs the negatives. Fish such as Pacific wild-caught salmon, trout, halibut, cod, sole, and most other whitefish are acceptable when eaten in moderate quantities. Swordfish, mackerel, shark, tuna, and tilefish are highly contaminated with mercury and should be avoided (see Note, page 251).

BEANS AND LEGUMES

The wide variety of beans and legumes available include adzuki beans, black beans, fava beans, garbanzo beans, kidney beans, lentils, lima beans, mung beans, navy (white) beans, peas, pinto beans, and soybeans. They are high in protein but also high in starch, which converts to sugar in the body. Therefore it's best to eat only small servings so you don't feed candida and cause inflammation. Legumes are also high in lectins (proteins that bind with carbohydrates), which can damage the gut lining and create leaky gut. Adzuki and mung beans are higher in protein than the others, so it's okay to eat slightly larger portions of these. Because of the starch and lectin content, I recommend avoiding beans and legumes completely for the first three months of your candida-cure diet.

In the U.S. soy is overprocessed and overconsumed and, in most cases, genetically modified. Since there is still much controversy about whether eating it is good or bad for you, I do not recommend eating it in any form, including whole soybeans, tempeh, tofu, soy milk, and soy protein isolate, which is found in protein powder and protein bars. The only soy that is permissible on the candida-cure diet is Bragg Liquid Aminos, which is an unfermented, non-GMO soy sauce.

To remove phytic acid from beans to help with assimilation and avoid flatulence, soak organic beans overnight, discard the water, and cook the soaked beans in fresh water. Prepare beans with one or more of the following herbs and spices for optimal digestion and taste: cumin, clove, caraway, dill, fennel, sage, thyme, onion, oregano, ginger, garlic, rosemary, tarragon, turmeric.

VEGETABLES

Organic vegetables are loaded with phytochemicals and micronutrients that are needed by the body to help it regenerate. Because vegetables have alkalizing properties, they also help reduce acidity in your body, which reduces inflammation. Ideally, 60 percent of your daily diet should be vegetables.

Green leafy vegetables are nutrient-dense foods and contribute greatly to healing MS, so you need to consume them daily. Because of the nutrient loss in our soils, it is also advisable to take a green food supplement (see Supplementation section, page 342).

Culinary herbs such as oregano, thyme, basil, cilantro, parsley, rosemary, and sage have great healing properties. Make sure to include them in your meals whenever possible.

Lastly, don't forget to incorporate sea vegetables (such as arame, kelp, dulse, nori, wakame, and sea cabbage), which are rich in minerals, including iodine. Most of us are lacking in iodine, which is essential for optimal thyroid function. Sea vegetables also bind with heavy metals and radioactive toxins and move them out of the body.

FRUITS

Organic fruits have many beneficial vitamins and minerals that keep your body balanced, but you need to limit your intake because they are high in natural sugars, which can feed candida and thereby contribute to the progression of MS. Berries contain the smallest amounts of sugar, and the skins have beneficial antioxidant properties. Limit yourself to one fruit (or a small handful of berries) a day.

DAIRY

The popular consensus has been that eating and drinking dairy products is the best way to supply the body with calcium. As I discussed earlier, I disagree. It's more beneficial to get your calcium from organic plant sources that contain calcium, such as dark-green leafy vegetables, sesame seeds, almonds, broccoli, and carrots. These foods also contain trace minerals that will assist the calcium to enter your bones.

The pasteurization and homogenization of cow's milk chemically alter its mineral composition and destroy its nutrients. This processing makes the milk more acidic to the body, with the end result being the leaching of calcium from the bones. In addition to eating the vegetables, nuts, and seeds that are good sources of calcium, small amounts of unsalted organic butter, ghee, and raw goat and sheep dairy products (milks and cheeses) are acceptable on the candida-cure diet. However, I recommend that you do not eat the raw goat and sheep milk products until you have been on the diet for ninety days.

If you are a pregnant or nursing woman with MS and want to consume dairy during the first three months of the program, I suggest eating pasteurized goat and sheep products because they are usually not as altered or as congesting as cow products and are easier to assimilate. You should *not* eat raw dairy products (or raw fish) while pregnant or nursing. Another option is Goatein (Garden of Life), a high-potency goat dairy powder that is predigested so that lactose-intolerant individuals can consume it.

Vitamin D plays a critical role in immune function, and a deficiency of this vitamin is prevalent in those with MS. I do not recommend getting it from dairy sources, but rather from vitamin D_3 supplementation or pure cod liver oil (tested to be free of heavy metals and rancidity).

SWEETENERS

Sweeteners that are acceptable on your program and that you may eat for the rest of your life are stevia, lo han fruit extract, chicory root, and xylitol. You can use all of these in small quantities throughout your candida program and afterwards.

Stevia, an herb from South America, helps to balance blood sugar and therefore is beneficial when treating candida. Lo han (or luo han) is an extract from a very sweet fruit. It has zero calories and zero glycemic impact and can be used to bake with as well as to sweeten foods. Chicory root is a fiber that contains inulin, a prebiotic that stimulates the growth of good bacteria in the digestive tract. It does not raise blood-sugar levels and is low in carbohydrates. It can be used for baking. Xylitol, which I talked about in Chapter 4, is a carbohydrate, but since it is metabolized slowly, it doesn't increase sugar levels rapidly if eaten in small quantities. It has been shown to be effective in preventing and reducing bacterial infections in the mouth, sinuses, and ears. Make sure your source comes from birch bark (The Ultimate Sweetener from Ultimate Life) instead of corn.

RAW VERSUS COOKED FOODS

Since cooking destroys important enzymes that your body needs for digesting and assimilating foods, the more raw vegetables and fruits you eat, the more enzymes and nutrients your body will take in. However, if your digestive system is out of balance, you might find that initially you will have trouble digesting raw vegetables. If this is the case, take digestive enzymes and eat steamed or cooked vegetables for a while, and then gradually increase your raw food intake with each meal. Continue taking the enzymes as necessary.

FOOD COMBINING

Proper food combining involves eating either protein with vegetables, or grains with vegetables. It's also important to avoid mixing animal protein with grains at the same meal, especially for some people who have digestive problems. However, others find that eating a little protein along with grains at each meal, whether it's protein from an animal or a plant source, keeps both their blood sugar and energy levels more stable.

The answer for you lies in listening to your body. If you're hypoglycemic, meaning you have low blood sugar, you'll do best to start off your morning with protein and work your complex carbohydrates into your lunch or dinner meals.

Most people with MS have sugar imbalances and do best initially eating three meals a day that include a little protein and having a snack mid-morning and in the afternoon, as this keeps their metabolism and energy levels balanced. If you are prone to excessive weight loss, however, eat only three meals a day and avoid snacking in order to slow down your metabolism.

FOOD ALLERGIES

The best cure for food allergies and intolerances is abstinence. Reactions to certain foods may include itchiness, hives, rapid heartbeat, fatigue, constipation, diarrhea, canker sores, gas, bloating, headaches, or a worsening of your MS symptoms. If you suffer from allergies or food sensitivities, eliminate trigger foods for at least one to three months to get rid of allergic reactions.

The most common trigger foods are those I mentioned earlier: milk, citrus fruits, chocolate, eggs, sugar, nightshade vegetables (tomatoes, peppers, potatoes, eggplant), soy, gluten (barley, kamut, oats, rye, spelt, triticale, white flour, wheat), peanuts, MSG, and corn. Of course it's possible that you may be allergic to other things as well.

After abstaining for three months from the foods you are sensitive to, you can test them by adding them back into your diet one at a time. Only reintroduce those foods that are acceptable on the candida-cure diet. Your body will tell you if it likes them or not. If you react, you know to stay away from those foods or to eat them in moderation only.

Keeping your diet varied is another way to avoid allergic and intolerance reactions. There are plenty of choices in each food group to ensure you are not eating the same thing day after day. As the saying goes, "Eat a rainbow of colored foods every day."

WATER

F. Batmanghelidj explains that the brain is 85 percent water and says: "Next to oxygen, water is the most essential material for the efficient working of the brain. Water is a primary nutrient for all brain functions and transmission of information."[1] This means that your body needs more water if you're to think and act rationally.

If you notice that your urine is a dark color, this indicates that you are dehydrated. As I said in the last chapter, the ideal amount of purified or filtered water to drink each day is one half of your body weight in ounces. So if you weigh 150 pounds, you need to drink 75 ounces, or a little over nine eight-ounce glasses of water. To make this easier to do, drink six ounces— a little less than one cup—every waking hour until you go to sleep. Don't let yourself get to the point of feeling thirsty. Drinking more water can eliminate a number of symptoms, including headaches and other bodily pains.

Distilled water and reverse osmosis water are good drinking waters, but they leach minerals from the body. So if you drink them, make sure to take your vitamin and mineral supplements daily. Sparkling mineral water in small amounts is acceptable as a soda replacement, but only if it's natural and the carbonation has not been added to it. One of the only true natural sparkling mineral waters is Gerolsteiner from Germany. Unsweetened electrolyte waters, such as Smart Water, are acceptable only after an exercise workout of more than an hour. Do not drink them continually throughout the day.

The best way to ensure that you are getting clean and purified water is to buy your own filtration system. I don't recommend most bottled waters because manufacturers are not regulated and you don't really know what you're getting. Also, plastics leach chemicals into the water that disrupt the endocrine system. If you do buy bottled water, look for a company that tells you how the water has been purified, or find a brand that states on the bottle how the water has been processed, such as through reverse osmosis. If this information is on the label, you have some assurance of the water's purity.

Sodas, coffee, iced tea, and fruit juices are not substitutes for water, but herbal teas can be.

HERBAL TEAS

Herbal teas count as water, but because most are diuretics, you need to make sure to put minerals back into your body by drinking some purified water. Among the many therapeutically beneficial teas available, I suggest red clover, pau d'arco, dandelion root, rosemary, green tea (caffeinated or decaffeinated), chamomile, hibiscus, and mint. You can mix and match for desired flavor and effect.

JUICING

Juicing is a great way to nourish your body. Fresh vegetable juice that has had the fiber extracted will immediately fill your bloodstream with live enzymes, vitamins, and minerals. Juicing is also alkalizing to your body because it draws out acidic waste products.

Juicing correctly is important when you are using it as a health treatment. First, don't make more than eight ounces of fresh juice at a time. Drinking large quantities, such as sixteen to thirty-two ounces of carrot juice at one time, can do more harm than good because this is too much sugar for your system to handle.

Second, drink juice on an empty stomach, either an hour before a meal or two hours after a meal. Since the juice acts as a treatment for your bloodstream, do not drink it with a heavy meal. Third, drink your juice as soon as you make it. Many of the vitamins and minerals become oxidized within thirty minutes of being exposed to the air. Fourth, drink your juice slowly. Swish it around in your mouth to mix it with your saliva, and then swallow.

I recommend the Breville juicer, which can be bought online at www.amazon.com or in many local department stores. There are many books on juicing that you can use to find recipes you like. One of my favorites is what I call Vegetable Alkalizer Juice (see recipe on page 308).

The Vitamix food processor is a wonderful way to eat whole foods and to make soup. It is different than juicing in that it retains the fiber, and your digestive system has to break it down. Juicing discards the fiber, allowing the juice go directly into the bloodstream. Both methods are beneficial for nourishing your body.

RELAX AND ENJOY YOUR FOOD!

Despite the fact that there is contamination of our food supply at every level and it continues to escalate, it's important to maintain a healthy mind-set about the situation. Stay abreast of reports regarding the foods that are most toxic—GMO foods, fish from contaminated waters, and crops sprayed with herbicides, pesticides, and fungicides, etc.

Do your best to buy organic, antibiotic- and hormone-free products, and grass-fed meats. If you are able, grow your own organic vegetables and raise well-fed chickens. You can also lessen the toxic load by varying your food choices. For instance, there have been reports of arsenic being found in rice. Rather than forfeiting the benefits of organic brown rice, don't eat it every day, but mix it up by also eating other gluten-free grains like quinoa, millet, and buckwheat. When you eat in restaurants, make the wisest choices possible based on what you now know, and just bless the rest!

The key is not to get stressed out about every little thing

that might be in your food and then burden your body with more stress. Relax and enjoy as you nourish and restore your body with good foods and positive thoughts.

CHAPTER ELEVEN

ENVIRONMENTAL MANAGEMENT

Although you have little control over the environmental conditions in the geographical area in which you live, you can do much to neutralize toxicity in your home and office space. Do all you can to control your personal environment by cleaning your airspace; drinking purified water; using nontoxic cleaning and body-care products; and eating organic fruits, nuts, and vegetables, grass-fed, antibiotic- and hormone-free meats, and unfarmed fish. Let go of what you can't control and trust that the steps you are taking will be sufficient.

CLEAN AIR

One of the most important things you can do is clean the air in your home and work space. Air-purifying technology is rapidly changing, so do your research to see what best fits your needs.

Ionizers and filter systems are the two basic types of air purifiers on the market. Variations of ionizers are available: some put out only negative ions, others produce negative ions and UV waves, and some put out negatively charged ions and ozone.

HEPA filters have been around for a long time. These units collect dust and hair in the room where they're located.

The filters can be expensive to change, and they don't get rid of molds and chemicals.

With ionizers that put out negative ions, these negatively charged particles attach themselves to airborne debris and cause it to drop to the floor. Some units add ozone to the air. At high levels, ozone can be irritating to your upper respiratory system, but it's quite effective in neutralizing molds, odors, and chemicals. Ionizers that use UV light waves eliminate the risk of ozone irritation and are still effective in getting rid of chemicals and molds. Units that generate ozone should only be used in the living room—not your bedroom. They may irritate your lungs.

If you have many allergies, you may want to invest in a peak flow meter, which will help you identify which of the rooms or spaces where you spend time are causing you distress. You simply breathe into the meter and measure your breath-level capacity. In spaces that contain allergens, you'll find that your breathing capacity is lower. You can search the Internet to find sources for these meters.

The purifying unit I use in my bedroom is Aclare Air, which uses photocatalysis technology to oxidize odors, fungi, mold, and toxic chemical gases. At the same time, it settles dust and other large particles out of the air and reduces microorganisms such as bacteria and viruses. (See the Resources section for information on where to purchase.)

CLEAN WATER

Water, one of the scarcest and most contaminated natural resources on the planet, needs to be purified, filtered, or distilled in order to be safely consumed. Bottled waters are not the best source of clean water because the companies that bottle them are not monitored. The levels of heavy metals, chlorine, and fluoride in them may be just as high as those in tap water. Also, as I said earlier, chemicals from the plastic bottles leach into the water, especially when exposed to the sun on delivery trucks.

The best way to control the quality of your water is to buy a filtration system that hooks up to your faucet. Use a system that filters out chemicals, heavy metals, parasites, and bacteria. As with air-purifying systems, you'll find many choices on the market. Structured matrix and reverse osmosis systems, and those that use ultraviolet light with a carbon filter are effective (see Resources).

If installing a home unit isn't an option, choose bottled distilled water over tap water. Some health food stores have reverse osmosis machines that you can use to fill up your own bottles.

BALANCING ELECTROMAGNETIC FIELDS

The marketplace is filled with gadgets that claim to counter the effects of exposure to electromagnetic fields (EMFs) and frequencies. I have not come across products that I feel can neutralize those frequencies. A simple way to realign your own energetic field each day is to sleep with your head toward magnetic north and your feet facing south.

By limiting your exposure to cell phones, microwave ovens, Blue Tooth headsets, Wi-Fi (turn off when not in use), power lines, hair dryers, and other high-frequency devices, you will reduce some of the harmful impact of EMFs on your body. "Bluetube" headsets have an air tube that is designed to prevent radiation from reaching your ear when using your cell phone and may be effective in somewhat reducing EMF exposure. You can find sources for these on the Internet.

NONTOXIC CLEANING AND
BODY-CARE PRODUCTS

Health food stores, vitacost.com, iherb.com, and amazon.com carry a wide range of safe cleaning and body-care products that are free of toxic chemicals. Changing to less toxic products is a small step, but it will reduce some of the stress on your immune system caused by chemicals that are easily absorbed through the skin from hair-care, cleaning, and skin-care products, as well as cosmetics.

Make sure to Read the ingredients on labels carefully, as even "natural" products sometimes contain harmful chemicals.

CHAPTER TWELVE

STRESS BUSTERS

S tress is part of life. We are given many opportunities to work through challenging situations that help us to grow and to survive. If you have MS, stress has been a major cause of your condition. If left unmanaged, it will aggravate and accelerate the course of the disease and provoke exacerbations. A diseased body cannot rejuvenate itself or create new cells when it's in a constant state of stress. Therefore it's important to find outlets to alleviate your stress through activities such as exercising, breathing, meditating, journaling, reading, visualizing your body as healthy, watching movies that make you laugh, getting out into the sunshine, and being in nature.

EXERCISE

Exercise is essential to rid your body and mind of distress, to keep your circulation flowing, and to maintain muscle tone. Exercise also releases endorphins, hormones that elevate your mood and help relieve pain.

To speed up your healing, it's essential to keep your circulation optimal so that toxins move out of your body. As I explained in Chapter 9, your lymphatic system plays a major role in removing this waste, but it requires exercise and other external stimulation to do its job. Exercising doesn't mean having to go to the gym every day and lifting heavy weights. You don't need to work that hard to keep your body toned. Your stage of MS will determine how active you can be. Walking, swimming, isometric exercises, tai chi, qigong, and yoga are excellent. Yoga and isometrics alone can be enough to stop muscle atrophy, or wasting. Yoga is also highly beneficial because it combines physical strengthening and toning with deep breathing.

Exercising three to five days a week is usually enough for almost everyone. If you are wheelchair bound or have limited mobility, isometrics are beneficial and easy to do. You basically tighten and hold each muscle group for five seconds, exhale while still holding the muscles tightly, and then release. Work up to holding each muscle group for thirty to sixty seconds. You can find many books on isometrics by searching www.amazon.com.

Angle therapy is also beneficial for those who are not ambulatory. For five minutes twice daily, lie on a bed or any flat surface on which you can elevate your legs above your heart and support your feet either against a wall or on a chair. You may also have someone hold your legs up—they don't have to be high above your heart, just high enough so that blood flow is moving from your feet and legs toward your head. This mechanically moves stagnant blood from your lower extremities.

BREATHING

Breathing is vital for alleviating stress, and its value is not to be underestimated or taken for granted. Focused, centered breathing calms down your mind, brings oxygen into your brain and cells, and releases poisons from the body.

Many of us are constantly running around taking care of endless tasks, never stopping to quiet our minds. This tends to create shallow breathing, from the chest up, rather than abdominal breathing, which engages the diaphragm and allows you to take in oxygen more fully. When you breathe this way, the abdomen expands on the inhale. So go outside, or sneak into the bathroom, or lie on your bed, or close your office door and breathe—deeply. Take time out for yourself and do this for a couple of minutes four times a day.

Pranayama breathing is an ancient Eastern practice of breathing that can accelerate healing and neutralize stress. You can learn how to practice this method by doing some research on the Internet. It's worth investigating.

MEDITATION

Meditation helps you to still your mind. It can relax you and thereby relieve mental and emotional stress, which is crucial for creating a strong immune system. Scientific studies have shown that meditation can create a state of relaxation in the body that is the opposite of the fight-or-flight stress response.

Meditation is not just a suggestion; I feel it is as mandatory for your healing as eating a healthy diet and detoxifying your body. Although meditation is an easy technique, it's often challenging to get started because it's also easy to find excuses not to sit still for five to twenty minutes a day. But the benefits make it worth the practice, and once you get into the habit, you may start looking forward to this time of silence and peace.

There are many forms of meditation, and the practice you choose depends on what feels right for you. In general, meditation is a way to retreat from the outside world and enter the world of your inner being. Here you can observe your thoughts and feelings as they arise and begin to release them. At first you might be amazed at the torrent of thoughts and sensations you experience. Don't be concerned. This is natural—they've always been there; you've just never been still enough to notice them. With continued practice, you may find that a peaceful spaciousness takes their place.

Start by meditating five minutes a day and build up as you are able. Here are some suggestions for simple techniques to get you going:

Sit in a comfortable position with your spine upright and your legs crossed (or in the lotus position), if possible. You can also lean against the headboard of your bed or sit on a chair or sofa with your feet flat on the floor. Close your eyes, and begin by taking some deep breaths. Silently repeat a mantra over and over in your mind to help you get into a relaxed state. This can be a syllable such as OM, or one word such as *one, now,* or *love.* Or, with eyes closed, look up and focus on your third eye (or inner eye), which is located just above and between your eyebrows. Another technique to slow down the mind is to gaze at a candle or at a spot on the wall in front of you. As you meditate, follow the natural rhythm of your breathing, allowing each inhale and exhale to take you deeper and deeper into relaxation.

Allow yourself to drift and float. If conscious thoughts keep flooding your mind, allow them to float by like the stock numbers on a ticker tape or clouds in the sky. It's okay if your conscious mind is overactive. The key is not to grab onto the thoughts and give them energy. Just see them float on by. Over time, you will become more proficient at letting your mind slow down.

During your meditation, allow yourself to be filled with the silence and to feel connected to all that is. Near the end of your meditation, visualize and feel your body as healthy. See and feel golden-white light from above entering through the crown of your head, healing and repairing every cell, organ, and tissue in your body. Breathe in the light, and exhale all pain, stress, and negativity. See your brain and spinal cord filled with the golden-white light.

Moments of stillness can bring forth the insight you need to help you move forward on your healing journey. The goal is to bring the equanimity of your meditation into your life by mindfully observing your thoughts, feelings, and reactions in everyday situations. The more you are able to do this, the easier it will be to transcend old patterns of negativity and fear because you will be in the "now" moment—your place of power. Stilling the mind through meditation strengthens your relationship with your higher self, whose innate wisdom can guide you to create health and balance in body, mind, and soul.

If you would like to receive more instruction on meditation, you might consider joining a meditation class in your local area. It's important to understand that simultaneous with meditation, it's helpful, if not necessary, to also work on your psychology and emotions by seeing a therapist or hypnotherapist, or by using an emotional clearing technique such as the one I describe in Chapter 13. When you practice meditation, "hidden," or suppressed, emotions and issues often arise, so get extra help if you feel you need it.

BASK IN THE SUNLIGHT

Getting just fifteen to twenty minutes of sunlight each day will nourish you with the vitamin D your body needs to absorb calcium and other minerals. Sunlight also promotes a positive, optimistic, and healing outlook. When outside, make sure that at least 20 percent of your skin is exposed, with your hands and face accounting for only 5 percent. If you're going to be out in direct sunlight for more than thirty minutes, put on sunscreen with an SPF of no more than 15. Higher SPFs contain higher concentrations of toxic chemicals. One natural sunscreen that I like is Keys Solar Rx. Another good brand is Sierra Madre Sun Cream, which is SPF 30, but completely natural.

GIFT YOURSELF

Spoil yourself. Getting healthy means honoring yourself first. Indulge in a massage once a month—or more often. Massage helps to move waste and tension from your body. Treat yourself to lunch and a movie. Go shopping and buy yourself something special to wear, or another great book to read, or a new tool for your hobby.

HOBBIES

Whether you're interested in crafts, photography, or just reading mystery novels, a hobby allows your mind to slow down, as it does in meditation, because you are focusing on one thing. The enjoyment you gain from hobbies helps to keep your body in balance. If your mobility is limited, create new ways to keep your mind active and focused. Try crossword or jigsaw puzzles, for example.

FAMILY AND FRIENDS

Enjoying social activities and "play" with family members, children, and friends is a positive way to take your mind off being sick. Make sure to laugh as much and as often as you can. Laughter releases endorphins, those beneficial chemicals produced by the brain that help you feel good and support your healing. Hugs are great too. At least once a day, share a hug with a loved one, including any animal friends. The key is to not isolate yourself, because that may add to feelings of despair and hopelessness.

JOURNAL WRITING

Writing, without self-editing, is a helpful way to relieve stress. It also gives you greater awareness and understanding of the suppressed thoughts, feelings, and beliefs you may be harboring that can negatively affect your health. Writing without judgment is important so that you express your true feelings. You can even rip up and throw away what you write, making this a cleansing process of acceptance and release.

GET IN TOUCH WITH EARTH'S MAGNETIC FIELD

You can use the earth's gravitational pull to neutralize stress. It's easy—try hugging a tree. Hug one for thirty seconds and feel the tension run down and out of your legs into the earth. When I started hugging trees, it took me a few months to stop looking around to see if anyone was watching me and thinking I was a nut. Feeling self-conscious will only create more stress, but give it a try and see if you can get beyond it.

You can also get in touch with the earth's gravitational pull by planting your bare feet on the grass or sand, or by putting a blanket on the grass or sand and lying on it stomach down. You'll feel your stress melt away.

ACUPUNCTURE, CHIROPRACTIC, AND
CRANIAL SACRAL THERAPY

These three therapies can be quite beneficial to add to your wellness plan. Acupuncture is a traditional Chinese medicine technique that uses hair-thin needles to activate energy flow (Chi) in the body and remove blockages. It has been effective in balancing hormones, increasing circulation, and alleviating stress and even pain.

Chiropractic therapy consists of spinal manipulation that adjusts the vertebrae. It is important to keep the spine in alignment to make sure discs are not subluxated, or compressed, which causes nerve compression and interferes with blood flow and the optimal flow of cerebrospinal fluid.

Cranial sacral therapy is a gentle, hands-on method of enhancing the functioning of the cranial system, which consists of the soft tissues and cerebrospinal fluid that surround and protect the brain and spinal cord. Practitioners apply gentle pressure to release restrictions and thereby help restore the central nervous system.

GET EXTRA HELP

Since it's crucial to alleviate chronic stress so that it doesn't destroy your health, you will need to invest in yourself by taking on the practices I've listed here. If you feel you need more help, get it. Seek out a therapist or hypnotherapist who works with stress reduction. Listen to CDs on the subject and/or find a trainer who will motivate and assist you to exercise. If you know that your stress levels are out of control, make the investment in reestablishing balance.

CHAPTER THIRTEEN

EMOTIONAL AND MENTAL FITNESS

Your emotional and mental strengths are your most powerful allies in beating MS. You can use your conscious and subconscious minds to help you heal by identifying and releasing the beliefs and emotions that are suppressing your immune system. To begin to do this, you must become more aware of the underlying patterns you have developed over a lifetime and delve more deeply into your relationship with yourself.

This may seem like a lot of effort, or something you just want to forget about. But the sooner you move out of denial and begin questioning your stored negative beliefs and emotions, such as fear and anger, the more quickly you can release them and arrive at a point where you truly feel that your past is a thing of the past.

It's easier said than done, because at this stage of your life you may not be conscious of the ways in which your actions are rooted in your fear-based emotions. Cleaning your emotional house doesn't mean that you need to relive every awful experience from your past. Rather, it means looking for patterns and themes that are continuing to play out and create dysfunction in your current life.

WHAT YOU THINK IS WHAT YOU ARE

Whether or not you believe it, you have absolute choice over how you react to everything you think and feel. It's your choice whether you let the diagnosis of MS devastate you—or whether you decide to beat it. By becoming more aware and energizing positive thoughts and feelings, you can actually help restore your cellular health.

MS has a strong emotional core component of suppressed anger or rage and the devaluing of the self. So uncovering your core fear-based emotions and releasing them is essential to your healing process. The first step toward emotional and mental healing is to start looking at this disease as the result of denial. Ask yourself, "What am I not accepting?" This is what it takes to begin uncovering what you've been hiding under the rug or putting on the shelf—whether it's anger, sadness, abandonment, rejection, or fear.

Overcoming MS will be a test of learning how to reclaim your power. It's an opportunity for you to transform, and doing that means finding ways to release the emotional and mental baggage that's keeping your central nervous system ravaged. There are many forms of assistance available today to help you with this task, such as counseling, hypnosis, prayer, energy work, journaling, and art therapy, among others.

The second step is to ask yourself, "Do I believe my body can regenerate on a cellular level?" If your answer is no, it's not going to be possible, because your body responds to your beliefs. If you only casually entertain a new idea about being able to regenerate your body, this will not override an entrenched belief system that says the opposite and that you've been holding on to for years. While you will see improvement by just following the diet and taking an antifungal and supplements, complete transformation will happen only when you make it a daily practice to be healthy on every level—mentally, emotionally, physically, and spiritually.

Begin to pay attention to your thoughts, and choose to energize only those that support your well-being. When negative fear-based thoughts come up, acknowledge them immediately, and then give them permission to "go play outside."

The three most important steps you can take to manage your mind are accepting your negative thoughts; giving yourself permission to get rid of them; and then replacing them with positive thoughts or a neutral action, such as taking a deep breath, drinking a glass of water, or refocusing on your work task.

HOW TO REACH YOUR SUBCONSCIOUS MIND

As mentioned in Part Two, we act and react from our subconscious mind. It's a storehouse of beliefs and habits that have been repeatedly reinforced. The secret of reaching the subconscious mind is to train it on a conscious level through focused speech and repetition. The two most powerful ways to accomplish this are through hypnosis and speaking out loud using affirmations and prayer.

When you're unhealthy, it's important to change the imprint of illness that's been stored in your subconscious mind. You may be storing belief systems that need to be replaced, fear-based emotions that need to be eliminated, and negative thought patterns that need to be changed. Once you do this work, you will experience inner peace and health on all levels.

HYPNOSIS

Hypnosis is one of the quickest and most powerful ways to speak to your subconscious mind and to release and change belief systems, thoughts, and fear-based emotions. Unfortunately, hypnosis still has many negative connotations attached to it. There's nothing scary about it once you understand how it works.

Hypnosis is simply a technique that uses deep relaxation and focused concentration. That's it. You don't need to fear that you'll be made to lose control or do something you don't want to do. If anything, you'll be more in control because hypnosis lets you slow down your conscious thoughts and become more aware of what's going on in the present moment. Once you're in a state of relaxation, your hypnotherapist has greater access to your subconscious mind and can offer suggestions that will assist your healing process. Your subconscious mind is always listening, but when you're relaxed and not consciously busy, spoken suggestions take greater hold. If you receive a suggestion that does not feel right to you, you will either ignore it or come out of the hypnotic state.

To understand hypnosis better, you need to understand that we're all electromagnetic beings. We generate measurable units of electrical energy. The brain can go into four states that have different energy frequencies, which are measured in cycles per second (Hz): alpha, beta, theta, and delta. In your conscious waking state, you are in beta, which produces a frequency of about 14 to 35 cycles per second. In beta mode, you're not 100 percent focused on just one thing; you're able to think, feel, and sense many things at once.

When you go into hypnosis, you drop down into the alpha state, at a brain wave frequency of only about 8 to 14 cycles per second, and the conscious mind is lulled. The hypnotic state is an altered state, not like dreaming or being awake, but very similar to the feeling you have when you're just waking up in the morning or when you're drifting off to sleep at night. It's in this state that the greatest learning takes place and also where the removal of fears, habit patterns, and emotions that don't serve you can occur. The two other levels of the mind are theta (present during deep meditation and light sleep) and delta (present in deep sleep).

We all go into hypnotic states every day. For example, you're daydreaming while driving on the freeway and all of a sudden realize you're at your exit, or you watch a two-hour movie and realize only when it ends that two hours have gone by. These are examples of being in a light state of hypnosis—the conscious mind has been either distracted or in focused concentration, which has allowed the subconscious mind to be in the driver's seat, so to speak.

Getting effective results from hypnosis requires two things. First, you need to have a strong desire to resolve the problem or issue. Second, you need to trust and feel a rapport with your hypnotherapist.

I've found that integrating hypnosis into my clients' treatments has been an extremely valuable tool in assisting their bodies to heal. I have my clients visualize and feel every cell, organ, and tissue repairing itself, and help them identify and release limiting belief systems and remove negative thoughts and emotions that are stored in their bodies at a cellular level. I basically open the door to the subconscious so that they can give themselves permission to heal. To make the work more effective, I record our hypnotherapy sessions so they can listen to them for the following twenty-one days as they are falling asleep and saturate their subconscious minds with positive suggestions.

Remember, thoughts create energy. If you think, imagine,

and feel a healthy body often enough, eventually you will become that vision and feeling.

SPEAKING OUT LOUD

Another effective way to reach your subconscious mind is to speak out loud. The vibrations of sound create frequencies that alter physical matter (think high-pitched note breaking a wine glass). Daily positive self-talk and affirmations spoken out loud will reinforce and expedite your healing process.

This simple concept of talking out loud is incredibly powerful, yet greatly overlooked. You may view speaking out loud to yourself as crazy, but I'm here to tell you that it works, especially when it comes to negative thoughts and fear-based emotions. Reflect on how the words of a song have affected you, or how a speech has moved you to tears, or how you have felt a sense of connectedness when engaging in a spoken prayer. It's the vibration of the words that cause you to feel. Affirmations, prayer, chanting, toning, and speaking out loud to yourself have one thing in common—they change your reality.

AFFIRMATIONS

Affirmations are statements or phrases spoken out loud that express a desired outcome. The act of repeating them helps to impress them on the subconscious mind, which responds to repetition. Therefore they're most effective when you speak them every day. Energize your affirmations by stating them with desire, belief, and conviction. I suggest repeating them seven times, but you can do more if you feel prompted. You may feel silly and embarrassed at first, but this will pass. Give yourself some privacy to make yourself more comfortable. Speak your affirmations in the car, in the shower, in front of the mirror in your bathroom, or when you take a walk.

As you say your affirmations day in and day out, you'll notice shifts taking place. Keep in mind that we've all had our subconscious minds programmed with negative affirmations verbalized by others, which we've believed and continued to repeat to ourselves. Now it's time to turn things around.

Stating what you envision to be desirable and the best possible outcome for yourself is not selfish. It simply means that you feel worthy of being all that you can be. A small side note: pay attention and be specific with your words and how you state what you are envisioning, because sometimes the thing you want most may come to you but in an unsettling way. Also, state your affirmation in the present tense, which affirms that what you are stating already exists. Say "I am . . . ," and not "I want . . . " or "I will have . . ."

Below are some examples of affirmations that you can use or modify. Part Four contains more examples. Don't be afraid to make up your own. You know better than anyone else what you need in order to move through your challenges.

Examples of Affirmations

- I am whole and complete in myself, my life, my work, my purpose.
- I am patient and tolerant. I accept what is.
- I love, accept, respect, trust, and honor my body and myself unconditionally.
- I am worthy because I exist. I exist; therefore I am worthy.
- Every day in every way I am better and better. Every day in every way I am healthier and healthier.

NEUTRALITY

I speak of being neutral in the sense of observing your life circumstances without judgment and without feeling a negative
emotional charge. In this way, you are better able to deal with
people and situations over which you have no control. You are
also protected from taking on others' negative energy because
that energy no longer finds resonance within you.

Neutrality is not something you can will to happen. Achieving this state requires releasing your fear-based emotions. By
doing this, people and situations that would ordinarily trigger
emotional reactions based on past negative experience no longer upset you.

Take the example of a woman who was sexually abused as
a child. The first step is for her to become aware and acknowledge that she's still carrying fear-based emotions around this
issue. Next, she needs to give herself permission to accept and
release the feelings of anger, violation, and sadness that she has
experienced. The final step is for her to work with her subconscious mind by using affirmations or hypnosis to replace these
fear-based emotions. Meditation and other emotional healing
techniques can also be of value in letting go of these old hurts
and fears.

The key is for this woman to release these feelings, which
will remove the emotional charge from the memory. By doing
this, she will be able to look back on her abuser and the experience with emotional neutrality and operate from a place
of freedom in the present. This takes a tremendous amount
of courage. Letting go of the anger might even allow her to
forgive or feel compassion for her abuser, and to begin to see
from a higher vantage point what she needed to learn from
that experience.

Every negative or traumatic event in your life can become either an opportunity to grow—or a prison in which you feel trapped.

NO LONGER A VICTIM

Another point to keep in mind when examining your emotions is that no one can "make" you feel anything. You have a choice about how you emotionally respond to people and circumstances.

When you think that other people make you feel something, you give away your power. For instance, if a man walks by you on the street and spits in your face, it's your choice whether you get angry, laugh, or remain neutral. People find it easier to assign blame to others for their challenges, but this only sets up a vicious cycle of being a victim.

Being codependent also keeps you victimized. In this scenario, you put others' needs before your own, thinking it's your responsibility to help or fix them. In a codependent relationship, even though you are giving, the unconscious motivation is to get something in return, whether it's love, acceptance, or just having someone who needs you. Eventually, you may end up drained because you're not taking care of you.

Do not give your power away. Instead, get in touch with it by accepting that you are the only one responsible for your happiness, and for your emotions. Be aware of the emotions that arise within your relationships and recognize where they're coming from. Notice if there are patterns that keep repeating in your life, and then deal with those issues using the Emotional Freedom Technique (described below) or another form of therapy, if necessary.

Taking responsibility for your emotions without blaming another—and doing the work necessary to release these stressful emotions—will help you to arrive at that place of neutrality. From there, you can choose appropriate actions that serve your highest good and the highest good of the other. Learn to feel confident in setting boundaries. This will help you to be calm and at peace when dealing with the difficult behaviors of those close to you.

HOW TO MOVE OUT OF FEAR AND ANXIETY

How can you heal your body if you're trapped in fear? You can't. Moving out of fear means having the courage to accept its presence, but also finding ways to move forward and beyond it. Because we have been conditioned by parents and society to live our lives in ways that keep us in bondage, it sometimes becomes necessary to give ourselves permission to cancel our former "contracts" and open the door to new ways of being. Once you give yourself permission to be free of fear, you are in a position to follow up with actions that support that choice.

Learning to move out of fear takes diligence and courage. Courage is the bravery and fortitude that enables you to move through situations even in the face of your fear. Diligence is the tenacity to work through a fear each time it comes up until it is gone.

The easiest and quickest technique to alleviate fear is to speak out loud. Address your fear directly, out loud, instead of trying to push it or your thoughts about it away. Speak to it as if it were a person. Let the fear know that you see it and that you don't want it sneaking up on you anymore. But accept it—don't deny it—when it does show up. Next, affirm that you're in control and that you won't let the fear dominate you. Give yourself permission to release it. Then replace it with what you want to feel that is positive or neutral.

For example, let's look at a woman who's afraid to drive on the freeway. As she approaches the freeway on-ramp, her heart starts to race, her palms sweat, and she has trouble breathing as her fears of getting into an accident surface. What she needs to do is immediately take a deep breath and speak out loud to her fear: "I see you trying to sneak up on me, but I'm not letting you in. I accept that I'm terrified to get on the freeway, but I'm not going to play into you right now. I'm in control. I refuse to give you any power. I give myself permission to release all this fear. I am now making a choice to think and feel differently." Then she needs to take a deep breath and exhale all the fear into the atmosphere, telling herself over and over again, either out loud or in her mind, "I'm confident and calm as I drive on the freeway."

Addressing your fears out loud instantly puts out the flames that are feeding them. This technique takes practice and conviction, but it's worth it because you will feel the results. Determination followed by positive action can turn negative spirals into positive outcomes. The key is to be persistent in retraining your thoughts and feelings and to keep telling yourself that you, not your fears, are in control.

In Chapter 7, I explained that there are two primary emotions—love and fear. Choosing to overcome your fears is an act of love toward yourself, and choosing love in all of its manifestations is your way out of fear. Making that choice does not mean you will never feel fear again. There are layers and layers of it that have accumulated throughout your lifetime, and it is an ongoing process to get to the bottom of it. Practices such as visualization, hypnosis, using the I Can Be Fearless app (see Resources) and the Emotional Freedom

Technique are powerful ways to help you move through fear permanently.

EMOTIONAL FREEDOM TECHNIQUE

Another tool you can use to deal with stubborn negative emotions is the Emotional Freedom Technique (EFT), developed by Gary Craig. This modality draws on theories from Thought Field Therapy (founded by Dr. Roger Callahan), acupuncture, neuro-linguistic programming, and energy medicine.

The practice involves focusing on an emotional issue and repeating a positive affirmation while simultaneously tapping on points on the upper body that correspond to acupuncture meridians, or nerve channels. Tapping is a quick and beneficial way to release and neutralize fears, phobias, traumatic memories, anxiety, stress, addictions, etc. It can remove deep-seated subconscious beliefs and the emotions attached to them.

The theory is that these emotions result from a disruption in the body's energy system, which may have been caused by a traumatic event or upset. This "stuck" energy manifests as physical reactions such as a jittery stomach, tight shoulders or jaw, racing heart, and sweaty palms when the painful memory is triggered. For example, if you almost drowned when you were a child, you may have a fear of water, and every time you approach a large body of water, your heart races like crazy and you break out in a cold sweat.

Tapping helps balance the nervous system by clearing the blocked channels and getting the energy flowing again. Each point is the end of a nerve channel. Since there is no easy way to know which nerve channel is holding a particular emotion, all the points are tapped, except in the abbreviated version described below.

Before tapping, you simply bring the emotion, pain, addiction, or traumatic memory to your awareness and briefly gauge how it feels. As you tap, you will feel the emotion clearing. Sometimes it takes only one session of tapping; other times you will need to repeat the process to let go of the emotion attached to a particular issue. You cannot overdo tapping. As you clear negative emotions and erroneous beliefs, you will become freer to find new and different ways to respond to people and situations in your life.

Abbreviated Tapping Technique

I have experimented and found an effective shortcut for the tapping technique. Instead of tapping on several points on the body, you just need to tap on the side of your left hand.

When you are feeling a negative emotion that you can't move through, the basic instruction is to create an affirmation that defines the feeling and also states that you unconditionally accept yourself in spite of it. Here's an example of an affirmation you could use: "Even though I am terrified of having MS, I deeply and completely accept myself." The statement allows the feelings to be present without resistance, and the tapping moves through the energy blocks to restore the flow of energy.

Bring together the fingertips of your right hand, and as you say the affirmation out loud, tap your fingertips against the side of your left hand—the fleshy part right underneath the bottom of your pinkie finger. Repeat the affirmation and tap until you feel the emotion dissipate. You might need to do this several times a day until it leaves.

Use the same format to phrase your affirmation any time you use this technique: "Even though I [clearly describe the feeling], I deeply and completely accept myself." Don't be shy with your adjectives and in expressing what you are feeling. The more you are honest with yourself and give yourself permission to accept your beliefs and emotions, the easier you can move through fear, anger, guilt, shame, etc.

More Examples

"Even though I am angry and hate my body, I deeply and completely accept myself."

"Even though I feel guilty about past choices, I deeply and completely accept myself."

"Even though I feel humiliated and weak because others have to take care of me, I deeply and completely accept myself."

Tapping is an excellent tool to use to improve your emotional and mental health, which can have a big impact on your physical well-being. Like anything else, if you use the practice only once, it is a novelty. The more you integrate this technique into your healing program, the more you will feel the benefits. To learn more about this process, search the Internet or look for books on www.amazon.com.

WHAT DO YOU WANT TO CREATE?

Each of us is a painter. Every day you use your palette to make choices that add colors and shapes to your life—or subtract them from it. Whether you want the responsibility or not, you are in control of your choices and actions, and you're the only one who determines the kind of minute, hour, day, week, and year you will experience. What picture do you want to paint? When you embrace your power and recognize that you orchestrate each day, you can begin to paint the colors and shapes that make you think and feel healthy.

When you stop and examine how your reality is created, you can see that everything originates from a thought, a fantasy, or a belief and is then followed up with emotion and/or action. Remember that you don't need to accept every single thought that goes through your mind and act on it. If you see your thoughts as clouds floating across the sky of your mind, just as you do in meditation, and don't latch on to them or emotionally react to them, you are freer to paint a more beautiful life. You are freer to create the moods and behave in ways that truly serve you best.

Your subconscious mind works diligently to make sure you become precisely the person you unconsciously believe yourself to be. So be sure that when you speak out loud, you only energize words that are positive and supportive of yourself and others. Likewise, only entertain and energize thoughts that are positive and creative. Emotions are certainly not all fear-based, so choose feelings such as joy, love, and excitement and make them part of your daily experience.

When you operate from love instead of fear, you create rather than destroy. Though it may seem that your mind, filled with negative fear-based thoughts, is against you, it really isn't. Rather, you are simply being tested—being given an opportunity to rise to the occasion, embrace your power, and paint the picture of your choice.

Living without fear is the greatest freedom you can experience. You'll know that you've moved past your fear when you face that old situation again but you no longer feel an emotional charge from it. You're neutral. By diligently using the tools and practicing the techniques that you feel are right for you, you'll reach the other side of fear with confidence. Trust, and give yourself permission to be successful in living a life free of fear, anxiety, and anger.

CHAPTER FOURTEEN

YOUR SPIRITUAL SELF

W e're seldom aware of the intangible and outdated beliefs that rule our lives. For example, you may believe MS is incurable, but this is not a law chiseled in stone. This kind of negative internal message will keep you enslaved in a diseased body. But you can change your beliefs.

On the spiritual level, this means gaining healing power from a relationship with a deeper part of yourself. Acknowledging your spiritual self means realizing that it too needs to be fed each day. You can do this by taking time for yourself in solitude and opening up to that power called God, Spirit, Tao, or whatever you wish to call it. Journaling, prayer, meditation, chanting, and saying affirmations are all ways to expand your spiritual self. Leading a busy life and having to earn enough money to put food on the table can be a distraction, but don't let that be an excuse for not tapping into the tools that can change your life.

Begin to treat each breath you take as if it were your first and last, and as an opportunity to make a choice for the better. The more you connect with your spiritual self and live in the now moment, the more you will find ways to enjoy the journey of life, and the more you'll stop racing to reach a destination that never seems reachable.

YOUR HIGHER SELF

This powerful connection to God that resides within each of us is called the higher self. It is all-knowing and contains the answers and guidance you need to move forward. You already know it as that gut feeling you have, or the little voice you hear but often ignore and later say, "I should have listened." It's that place inside that you become aware of when you feel that something is "right." The more you connect with your higher self using the practices mentioned above, the more you'll be able to utilize your full capacity to heal. Sometimes, asking your higher self for assistance and letting go of any preconceived ideas of the mind is all that it takes to turn a challenge around.

To tune into your higher self, you need to be able to move out of your ego into a place of neutrality, openness, and observation. Easy to say, but challenging to do. Start by slowing down and taking time out for yourself each day. The reason meditation and prayer are wonderful ways to access your higher self is because you slow down into that space of stillness and nothingness that connects you to all that is.

The ego is necessary, but many times it keeps you stuck in judgment, blame, and fear-based emotions. When you are operating from your higher self, you detach from the chaos around you and move into a space of clarity and wisdom that lets you make more positive choices. You can step back from yourself and see your challenge against the backdrop of a realm in which there are no limitations and many options. This state of clarity, vision, and power can be scary, and you may find it easier to remain in your familiar conditions and environments even though they are self-limiting and keep you stuck. But you have so much more to gain by having the courage to move forward with your spiritual expansion.

The God force may not be tangible to you at the moment, but it's always there; you just need to believe in it and allow it in. Trust is the necessary ingredient to make the connection and feel that power.

TRUST

Trust means putting your confidence in someone or something you strongly believe will serve your best interests. Sometimes trust develops out of tried-and-true experience; other times it's based on a gut feeling or an inner knowing. Since we can never predict the future based on the past, there's always an element of faith in trust. The two go hand in hand.

Without trust in yourself, a guide, or a higher power, fear can take over and weaken and eventually destroy you. The law of attraction simply states that what you fear is what you will attract. Living without trust creates anxiety because you're always waiting for the other shoe to drop.

Trusting—knowing that there's something greater than you that's positive and always available to assist you—takes practice and means surrendering to that power, especially during times of challenge. If the word *trust* brings up resistance in you, move into a feeling of self-honor and compassion, as this is the fertile ground in which trust can bloom. Relaxing and accepting every part of yourself, including your negative emotions (as you do when practicing the Emotional Freedom Technique), will spark compassion. Let that compassion encompass your disease and the choices that brought you to where you are now. As you gain more clarity, peace, and strength in this process, you will have greater trust in yourself and in the power that is leading you and enabling you to take the necessary steps to overcome your condition.

When it comes to your beliefs—whether about health, relationships, money, or any other aspect of your life—you have, at some level, placed your trust in them to give you what you want. Yet when you examine your current situation and it doesn't match up with the picture you had in mind for your life, it's time to question those beliefs because they are the foundation of who you are. If you're unhealthy, it is certain that you have been buying into beliefs that are working against you and creating imbalance.

BELIEFS

The secret to making your beliefs work for you is to consciously become aware of them and to then question those that are outdated and limiting. Sit down and ask yourself what you honestly believe about health, money, your self-worth, career, relationships, and the other aspects of your life. Begin to challenge everything, from the mundane to the unconventional, such as whether you can regenerate your body on a cellular level. Break apart each belief to get to its core by asking yourself these questions: "Where did it originate? Why am I carrying it? Does it serve any purpose now? Is it productive and positive or is it damaging to me in some way? And if so, how?"

This exercise may seem tedious, but it is a life tool that can help you overcome any challenge, including transforming an unhealthy body into a healthy one. Take this process on not as a chore, but rather as an exploration into the depths of who you truly are. In Part Four, you will have the opportunity to examine and write down the beliefs you hold in many areas of your life. Aside from revealing hidden motivations that you were unaware of, writing them down allows you to refer back to them later so you can spot them if they pop up again. It's a good idea to repeat this exercise periodically, because as you uncover the more apparent beliefs, you will discover that there are layers and layers of even more subtle beliefs residing deeper in your subconscious.

As I've said before, it's your interpretation of a diagnosis or an illness that determines whether it will cripple you or if you will turn it around. At times, you may find it hard to believe that you have that much power, but you do. You have the power to change your reality at any time. If you believe that MS has come upon you because of something outside your control, then you will have no power to overcome it. But if you accept that your lifestyle, habits, patterns, and thoughts have brought you to this point, then you have the power to let go of the disease and manifest health once again.

The body is inherently intelligent and knows exactly what to do to change and create health, but it needs your help. You must make the choice to be healthy by taking actions that create the environment your body needs to function optimally. It doesn't matter what anyone else thinks about how you are choosing to deal with your condition. You can challenge the establishment called "society" and "family" and still come out a winner. You have no control over how others perceive you, so why waste time trying to appease those around you when you're suffering? Learn to tune in to what you trust and feel. Walk to your own beat. Create new beliefs that feel right to you and allow you to live out your heart's desire.

CHANGING YOUR BELIEFS

You can intellectually grasp how to change a belief in a few seconds, but really integrating it and feeling it deeply takes time. It's important to keep a new belief in your consciousness and to uphold it each day. This takes perseverance and courage be-cause you are changing fundamental ways that you've operated in the past.

You may even find that you need to let go of unhealthy en-vironments and relationships. As you move through every day, the key is to honor what you now feel to be true. Soon that belief will become ingrained in you and influence your percep-tions, thoughts, and feelings.

GRATITUDE

Many MS sufferers are afflicted with buried anger. This is not something to be ashamed of—every illness has its own core issues that provide an opportunity to learn and grow. I have found that often there is resistance in people that stems from denial about the reality of their condition and its underlying causes. Know that moving into acceptance and feeling grateful for every experience, whether good or bad, will help your heal-ing progress more rapidly.

You might ask, "Why would I give thanks for a disease?" The answer is simple. Were it not for this experience, you would not be able to discover the truths that can set you free, not only from this disease but from ways of thinking and feel-ing that prevent you from being truly happy and at peace.

If you think that life or God has dealt you a bad hand, you will end up feeling bitter and resentful—states that are not conducive to health. On the other hand, if you accept your cir-cumstances with grace and gratitude and choose to grow from them, you are making a choice to be healthy.

Living a life of gratitude and grace is what I call the quintes-sential way of being. Acting with grace involves surrendering and allowing yourself to be guided from a higher vantage point than the ego, which thinks it always needs to be in control. Gratitude means accepting who you are and being thankful for what you have right now. It means being present and not hungering for what you don't have or projecting into the future with thoughts of what you need to be doing. The key is to relax and take one step at a time. Being grateful each day is the quickest way to allow more love, more health, and more joy into your life.

JOY OF THE SPIRIT

Being spiritual doesn't mean you have to be heavy and serious. On the contrary, it is your spirit that reminds you to connect with the child within, who loves to play and be joyful. Fun, joy, and laughter nourish every cell in your body by releasing healthy hormones that improve the functioning of your immune system.

Even in the worst health crises, you can find joy and laughter if you look for it. Laughter conquers any darkness and is a powerful tool for healing, as Norman Cousins demonstrated when he turned around a life-threatening disease with daily doses of Marx Brothers movies and *Candid Camera*. Laughter positively affects your cells by releasing endorphins. It also keeps you in touch with the now moment, which is always your place of power. In my case, my mother was the comedian who kept me laughing throughout my ordeal.

Allow the joyful spirit that you are to shine through more and more each day by creating new beliefs that are healthy, by being in the now moment and accepting what is, and by trusting the power of God to assist you with your challenge. Your higher self, your spiritual connection to God, is the unseen thread that weaves magic into your life each and every day—if you pay attention to it and allow it in.

CHAPTER FIFTEEN

YOU DON'T HAVE TO BE PERFECT

To heal MS, you need to commit yourself to a treatment plan. It's a challenge, but understand that you don't have to do everything perfectly. You'll find it easier to stay motivated and inspired in the face of fear and resistance if you keep in mind that there's always room for growth and you can only do the best you're capable of doing in the moment. I now believe this is the true meaning of perfection. So shift your belief about perfection from "I'm not good enough, so I must do everything perfectly to be accepted and validated" to "I love and accept myself as I'm growing and making progress and know there is room for improvement."

Trust that your healing will happen at a pace that feels right for you. Pay attention and recognize self-sabotaging behaviors, feelings, and thoughts when they show up, and replace them with those that are self-affirming: unconditional love, positive self-worth, self-tolerance, and acceptance of your individuality.

SELF-WORTH

When I ask MS clients, "Do you feel you're worth your existence?" they usually answer "No." Sometimes they even break down in tears as they recognize this sad reality. If your answer is "No" or "I'm not sure," you're sending out signals that will bring about great imbalance in your body and mind. Feelings of unworthiness make it impossible for you to transform your body and heal.

Unfortunately, most of us were raised to believe that our self-worth depends on acceptance by others, how much money we make, whether we're healthy or not, how we look, and so on. However, self-worth is based on our intrinsic existence, not on what we do or have. Since we are all composed of the same energetic substance as everything in the known universe, each of us is part of all that is—and therefore worthy. Whether your contribution to life is positive or negative depends on the choices you make, but your inherent worth is not in question.

Sometimes illness is a wall that people hide behind because they feel they aren't good enough and are unwilling to accept the value of their individuality. Each of us is unique, with skills, gifts, and contributions to share with the rest of the world. We all have a purpose in life, which is to learn and grow from our personal circumstances, whatever they may be. The truth is, you don't need to compare yourself to anyone or prove yourself to anyone.

Check in with yourself, question your beliefs about self-worth, and see if they're truly valid from where you stand today. Are they keeping you stuck in patterns of resenting yourself or feeling intense pressure to succeed? If so, you have a choice to release those old beliefs and take on new ones that will benefit you. When I finally embraced my worthiness based on my existence alone, I found peace, freedom, and renewed health. The same can happen to you.

SELF-ACCEPTANCE AND UNCONDITIONAL LOVE

Once you've established your self-worth, you can begin to open the door to unconditional love. What does this mean? It means accepting yourself on all levels and loving yourself for who you are. When you operate from a place of unconditional love, you are self-compassionate and self-nurturing when you make mistakes. Embracing unconditional love is the most powerful way to mend any divisions between your body and your mind.

Few of us ever learned total self-acceptance when we were growing up. Unfortunately, we are products of negative conditioning and have come to associate receiving love and approval with "good" behavior. Like the rest of the human race, you've been programmed since birth with messages and beliefs that are stored deep within your subconscious mind, perhaps telling you that you're not good enough, or that you've "failed," or that you "should have" or "could have" done this or that.

If you haven't stopped to question these negative and self-defeating messages, you're no doubt still playing them out in your adult life. The end result is that you are extremely self-critical. When you continue to treat yourself like a bad dog that learns only when it's beaten, your body responds by creating toxins and eventually shutting down. You become your own worst enemy by unconsciously looking for validation and acceptance through an illness.

This lack of unconditional self-love defeats your very core, your self-worth, and traps you in negativity and self-doubt. You lose touch with your true essence—the part of you that loves you no matter what experience you go through, the part of you that's your own best cheerleader and lets you know that you can do anything you desire.

Learning to treat yourself as your own best friend is an important ingredient of transformation. This may sound corny, but it's true. Think about how you treat yourself compared to how you treat your best friend. Whether you like it or not, you're in a relationship with yourself. That relationship can be positive or negative—it's your choice.

Cultivating a positive relationship with yourself requires patience as you diligently work on changing your beliefs. When you tear down the walls of judgment and fear through complete self-acceptance, you increase your self-esteem, confidence, and empowerment. By reaching out and grabbing your power, you can witness your body overcoming a so-called incurable disease and create success in every area of your life. You can't divorce yourself, so why not make the journey more enriching by becoming your own best friend and treating yourself with compassion, tolerance, courtesy, understanding, and unconditional love?

Self-acceptance creates the opening for something new to unfold within you. The first step is to accept who you are right now, in this very moment. This includes all your challenges and your shadow side, the part of you that contains the so-called negative traits. The simple act of accepting what you have been afraid to look at before because you thought it meant you were a bad person is freeing in itself.

When you don't accept what is, you are in a place of resistance. For example, if you refuse to be realistic about your current condition and you use crutches when you need to be in a wheelchair and then fall and break your hip, you are resisting what is. Rather than being honest and compassionate with yourself, you may find yourself in denial about the progression of your disease and repeat the same self-destructive actions until there are serious repercussions. Resistance keeps you stuck, makes you feel angry and impatient, and ultimately creates vicious cycles of mental, emotional, and physical pain and suffering that can last weeks, months, and even years.

The most important step that you can take toward self-acceptance is to stop beating yourself up and carrying around guilt that serves no purpose. Learn from your past experiences and realize you have the power to make wiser choices now. Self-acceptance lifts all burdens, leaving you with a wonderful feeling of freedom. (See Figure 15.1.)

From self-acceptance, you can move into a place of choice—the conscious choice to uphold your commitment to love yourself unconditionally. The goal is to become your own coach and to support yourself during good and challenging times alike. The fastest way to make that change is to pay attention and catch your self-defeating thoughts in action. Then immediately replace them with self-affirming statements.

Give affirmations such as "I love and accept myself and my body unconditionally" and "I am worthy." Speak out loud to yourself while looking in the mirror, and repeat these affirmations every day many times over. Express your affirmations with conviction by feeling them resonate in your solar plexus, located in the center of your abdomen. Soon you'll notice a shift in your self-esteem and confidence.

Also, when you feel you've made a mistake, observe your thoughts and see if you're engaging in self-critical inner dialogue. If you are, accept and acknowledge those thoughts and say, "Stop. I'm not going to engage in this. I'm tired of playing this game. Now, go play outside." Then replace those thoughts with positive or neutral ones. You want to get to the point where at times like this you are in the habit of telling yourself, "That's okay. Next time I'll do better" and "I can do it—I believe in myself." This technique is simple and effective when done repetitively. As you release the negative and energize the positive, you retrain your thoughts so they support you and create a new reality.

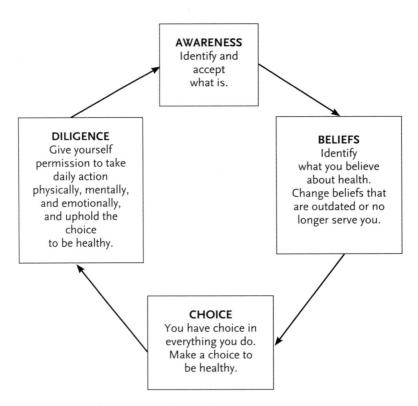

FIGURE 15.1. The ABCDs of Transformation

FORGIVENESS

Another essential ingredient of self-acceptance is forgiveness. It's important to spend some time forgiving those who have hurt you. When you do this, you are not applauding a person's actions, but are taking back your power by no longer engaging your energy in the emotions surrounding the event, such as resentment, anger, or hatred. By accepting what occurred, there is no longer a negative emotional charge surrounding the experience, but instead neutrality. From here, you are free to move into a state of forgiveness and go forward with the wisdom you gained from the experience. This will be an ongoing process throughout your life, as memories surface over time and as new opportunities arise each day to forgive those who appear to be harming you or others.

Most of all, you must forgive yourself—including the little child and the adolescent inside of you—for what you have done or think you should have done differently. Accepting every event in your past and knowing that there's no such thing as failure, only experience, will set you free. Recognize that negative and traumatic events from the past can be building blocks to a more positive future—if you allow them to be.

COURAGE AND TENACITY

I know that MS can be a very challenging condition, but dig deep for the courage and diligence to stick with a regimen, and trust that you're getting better every day. Staying committed to yourself does not mean monitoring, grading, and judging yourself. It means having a game plan and doing the best you can to stick with it.

BE HERE NOW

Staying in the now moment is essential to feel motivated. The past is over, so focusing on what you could have done will only weigh you down. Anxiety-filled thoughts about the future will only paralyze you more. The now moment is your place of power. Stay in today! Tell yourself: "Today I am stronger. Today I make better food choices. Today I have more compassion about my condition and myself. Today I am healthy!"

DON'T GIVE UP

Read this chapter over and over again whenever you start to feel discouraged and want to throw in the towel. Don't give up. (See Part Four, "Fear Busters.") Ups and downs are to be expected, so learn to ride the waves, which are common when healing MS. Remember that your central nervous system takes longer to heal than any other system in your body.

Even though it may take you just one moment of thought to realize you can heal, your physical body has a residual memory that responds more slowly. Cellular memory can change, but sometimes it behaves like a stubborn mule. If you're aware of this, you will have the strength to keep following the program and not give up because you think it's not working. Be patient and trust.

You don't have to be perfect to heal your body; you do need to be diligent and tenacious. However, on days when you just don't want to eat what you're supposed to or you can't get up enough energy to exercise, don't. Be sensitive to your needs. At the same time, be aware that it's easy to be lax and then claim that the program didn't work. You may very well experience moments of self-sabotage when you don't eat healthy or take your supplements, or you "fall down" in some other way. Be willing to love yourself even in those moments—and then get back on track. Each baby step equates to success because it brings you closer to your goal!

CHAPTER SIXTEEN

CLIENTS' STORIES

The following case stories are from clients who have MS and are healing. It has been an honor to assist and watch the courage, diligence, and growth of each and every one of them.

LINDA

BACKGROUND: often sick, diagnosed with Crohn's disease at 23, severe trauma to body at age 40 due to electrocution, allergies, high blood pressure, high sugar intake

SYMPTOMS UPON VISIT: numbness, tingling, weakness, spasticity, fatigue, stomach pain, using cane/walker and wheelchair

PHARMACEUTICALS TAKEN FOR MS: Copaxone (3½ years), Tysabri (3 years), steroids, Baclofen, Neurontin, Provigil

ANTIBIOTICS: took antibiotics often in adulthood and as a child

DATE OF FIRST VISIT WITH ANN: June 2010

From as early as my teen years, I had unexplainable issues with my body. My legs would give out on me, I would lose feeling in different body parts, or I would be overwhelmed by fatigue. These symptoms would come and go, so doctors could never figure out what was happening. At the age of 40, I was severely electrocuted, which left my body very damaged. Doctors told me I was lucky to be alive and that in time I would get better. But I didn't get better—I got worse. The little symptoms I had experienced for so many years now overtook my life. I could not feel my body most of the time. My legs, hands, and feet felt as though they were always burning. I went from taking long walks each day to not being able to walk at all at times, and the fatigue that was once just annoying became overwhelming.

I was sent from doctor to doctor, but none of them could tell me why I was getting worse from the accident. I have an aunt with MS, so I was familiar with the disease. My husband researched it further, and my symptoms matched all that he was reading about. We found an MS specialist, who confirmed I had it. Most likely the electrocution triggered my first full-blown MS attack.

I began taking Copaxone, which didn't stop the relapses that were now happening about every two months. My doctor wanted me to try the drug Tysabri as soon as it came out. I did much better on this medication. However, the drug could not be taken for more than two years. After three years my doctor said I had to stop, and I was placed on Rebif. I became very sick from this medication. I felt as though I had the flu all the time. I felt this was no way to live my life and began to look for a better way to fight MS.

When I was first diagnosed, I had Ann Boroch's book *Healing Multiple Sclerosis*. But being that I was a sugar addict, I wasn't willing to give up the foods that gave me great comfort. I didn't want to believe that I was actually feeding MS each time I ate my comfort foods! This time I looked at the book through different eyes. I had suffered greatly, had given up too many activities, and I no longer wanted to have to go places in a wheelchair.

I was now a grandmother and didn't want to be the grandma in the wheelchair. I wanted to run, play, and dance with my grandchildren. So I reread Ann's book. Meanwhile, the MS support group that I facilitated was looking for someone to come speak to our group about MS and nutrition. One member told me that she knew a man with MS who had been in a wheelchair, but after following the diet of a nutritionist, he was no longer in the wheelchair. I asked her to get the name of the nutritionist. When I was given the name Ann Boroch from the member of my group, I knew I wanted to talk with her to help me.

This was the best decision I had made! I met with Ann and began her diet, which I found to be much easier than I thought it would be. Within a few months my MS symptoms went away and I got my life back! I was able to do all the activities that I had not been able to do in years. I no longer needed daily naps just to get through a day. I went from being taken care of to taking care of others. I wanted to kick myself for not starting this diet when I first got Ann's book. All those years of suffering, pain, and loss could have been avoided.

OUTCOME: I have been relapse-free since starting Ann's diet two-and-a-half years ago. I have not once needed to use my cane, walker, or wheelchair. Since being on the diet, I no longer take meds for MS symptoms or disease-modifying drugs. And most importantly, I am the grandmother who runs, plays, and dances with her grandchildren. When I was able to walk through Disneyland with my three-year-old granddaughter, I knew that there was no food more important to me than the feeling I felt that day!

ANNE

BACKGROUND: childhood chicken pox, mononucleosis as a teenager, substance abuse, stresses (unhealthy long-term relationship and job losses), mercury fillings removed

Symptoms upon visit: pain, weak legs, balance problems, bladder dysfunction, spasticity, foot drop, migraine headaches

Pharmaceuticals taken for MS: Betaseron, Baclofen, Neurontin, Nortriptyline, 3 rounds of steroids in the 90s

Antibiotics: 10–12 rounds in lifetime

Date of first visit with Ann: August 2011

In December 1990, I received a very unwanted Christmas present. On the 26th, I got the diagnosis of multiple sclerosis. I didn't even know what it was, but it scared me. I was an active 28-year-old working full time, who liked to walk and bike around the neighborhood and hang out with friends. For the previous six months I had been experiencing numbness in my legs and trunk, balance problems, and leg weakness, which led me to see a neurologist at the request of my chiropractor. A second opinion confirmed the diagnosis after I had an MRI and other diagnostic tests (visual-evoked response, auditory, and pain stimulus tests).

During the next three years I had relapses about every nine months, for which I received steroids. I developed additional symptoms of bladder dysfunction, tingling sensations, spasticity, pain, optic neuritis, and Lhermitte's sign (electrical sensation down back when head bent forward). I was frequently fearful of the future, wondering what else was going to go haywire with my body. My doctor had started me on symptom-control drugs that helped some. In 1994 I began taking the interferon Betaseron—the first disease-modifying drug on the market. After starting Betaseron, I had no more relapses and my MS became stable for about ten years.

Around 2004, my MS started gradually getting worse. I was unable to grocery shop by foot, needed a wheelchair for long distances, and was having a harder time working. (I continued to work at a full-time job even after MS entered my life.) Essentially, everything was harder to do with the increased pain and leg weakness. By May 2011, my life was reduced to working and lying on the couch.

At this time, a friend of mine with MS told me how much her MS had improved and about all the activities she was doing. I asked her how she was able to do it and she told me about Ann's book, *Healing Multiple Sclerosis*. I jumped onto Amazon's site as soon as I hung up the phone and ordered the book. I read it straight through, practically nonstop. I have to admit I was overwhelmed at the idea of drastically changing my diet and taking a bunch of supplements, especially since this was during a chaotic time in my life due to the health crisis of a close family member. I sat with the idea for about two weeks, rereading the lists of foods to eat and not to eat and preparing mentally to begin my healing journey. I realized that there was not going to be a perfect time to start, and I knew that my MS was getting worse. I had nothing to lose and everything to gain by starting Ann's program. I made up my mind—I wanted a better life for my husband and myself.

I began by bringing the allowed foods in the house and eliminated one major item: coffee! I had been a daily coffee drinker since I was 18 and loved my coffee! After a few days I just jumped into the diet full-on and stuck to it. Reading ingredient labels became a new normal. I quickly learned that we are surrounded everywhere with "no-no" foods, and choosing to not eat them can be a challenge. (I sit literally three feet from the coffee maker at work and a counter that usually has cookies, donuts, pastries, bagels, cream cheese, and candy on it.) Whenever I'm tempted to veer off the diet and eat these kinds foods, I say to myself, "Nothing tastes as good as walking feels." As hard as it is to turn down certain foods, it is much harder to live with the ravages of MS.

As the months move along, I find that I don't want "no-no" foods very often anyway. I love the feeling I get from providing nourishing foods to my body and not feeding the MS. When I'm tempted, I think to myself that if I eat the wrong foods my healing will be slowed. I am also continuously motivated to eat the correct foods because it keeps my weight controlled. I dropped 22 pounds after starting the candida diet, and I feel much better because of it.

When I read the stories in Ann's book from the clients who said they eventually got off all their MS drugs, I was astonished. I could not imagine living with MS without my crutches called pharmaceuticals. I had been on various combinations of drugs for twenty-plus years. Ten years ago I got off all my drugs to prepare for pregnancy, but my symptoms were intolerable, so I got back on all of them. After starting Ann's program, I wondered if I would be able to get off them again, and if so, how would I know when? I decided that time would tell. Four months in, I had the confidence to wean off one pain medication since I was feeling better. By nine months into the program, I was off all MS pharmaceuticals. By doing Ann's program, my beliefs about how to treat my MS were changed—I knew that the drugs I was taking were not effective anymore.

During my healing journey, there have been many ups and downs—it is definitely not a straight line. I have struggled with this since the beginning and would be mentally crushed when I hit a valley after feeling so good for a period of time. I have to say that my family (spouse, mom, brother, in-laws) have been very instrumental in getting me through these times, reminding me that I am getting better and that healing will come. They remind me that I've had MS for twenty-two years, so it will take time to reverse it. I'm learning to be more patient with the healing process, but it's a work in progress. During recent months I've worked on trying to keep my anxiety about the healing process away, knowing that negative emotions only hinder the process. I've incorporated meditation into my routine, and I believe this helps me trust that full healing will occur at my body's pace.

I saw my neurologist two months after starting Ann's program. He has been my neurologist for ten years, so he knows my history very well. I wanted his approval of Ann's program, but was not sure what he would say. I knew I was going to keep on the program even if he did not approve. I have learned throughout the years that our bodies belong to us and ultimately it is our decision how we treat our illness. Ann's program felt right for me. I brought in her book, *Healing Multiple Sclerosis*, and informed him that this was the approach I was taking to deal with my MS. He did not voice an opinion about whether he thought it would work or not, but said that he did not see anything wrong with it and that his wife ate similarly.

At that time I was still on all my medication. As the months went on and I began to heal, I would inform my neurologist that I wanted to get off one and then another of my drugs, and he would instruct me how to wean off safely, never once telling me that I should not be doing it. He recently said that he applauds what I'm doing and even supported my discontinuation of Betaseron.

OUTCOME: I am still in the healing process and have a long way to reach complete reversal, but I have made great improvements in the past year: my walking is faster, smoother, and easier, and I am no longer using my wheelchair or WalkAide. I have less pain and weakness, improved balance, and am off all MS and other pharmaceutical drugs. I feel confident that I am on the road to MS reversal in my near future.

BIRGITTA

BACKGROUND: measles, mumps, chicken pox, scarlet fever, migraines, injured back/neck in car accident at 6, high blood pressure, sinusitis, skin problems

SYMPTOMS UPON VISIT: numbness, migraines, skin problems, sinus congestion

PHARMACEUTICALS TAKEN FOR MS: Avonex, Betaseron

ANTIBIOTICS: over 100 courses in lifetime

DATE OF FIRST VISIT WITH ANN: April 2008

I was diagnosed with MS in the fall of 2002. My children at the time were 11 and 14 years old, and together with my husband they were my very strong support group.

As one would expect, I was shocked, enraged, scared, and sad, among many other feelings. My symptoms at the time were left-side weakness, numb toes on my left foot, double vision, and an increasing feeling of dizziness. I am someone who, aside from migraines since I was 7, could probably be considered a very healthy and strong person. To say I was caught by surprise is putting it mildly.

After dealing with the very acute symptoms with IV steroids, I quickly got started on weekly injections of Avonex. At times I had to deal with some cold and flu symptoms on the night of and morning after the injection, though the most common side effect was headaches.

A couple of months after my diagnosis I started a ten-week Living Well with MS program at UCLA. It is a program designed to help you understand as much as possible about the illness, as well as give you an arsenal of skills to use. I was especially interested in the exercises and yoga to work on my balance. What really got my attention were the more spiritual aspects to help you deal with what could become a lifetime of illness. One thing that kept being brought to the forefront in our class was the fact that MS can be exaggerated when you are feeling stressed, so a lot of what we learned was how to best de-stress our lives. The funny thing is that I can get very busy and do many things at once, but I tend to seldom feel stressed. I attribute that to my personality.

Toward the end of the MS class, I wanted to figure out how emotional issues might be contributing to my condition. With the help of a very good therapist, I started to feel that my migraines for many years had been a sort of warning light telling me when I was overdoing and overcommitting in my life. Having never been someone who was afraid of hard work (born and raised on a farm in Sweden), I was always among that group of parents who volunteered to bake cupcakes, do the fundraisers, be the room parent, drive the carpool, do the field trip, host the party, etc. Along with a part-time job as a preschool teacher, I, like so many parents, had a very full schedule. I now came to the realization that it might be a very good time to start cutting down on my involvement. Of course, my getting sick had put an immediate stop to many activities, but I was starting to feel better and had planned on getting back into everything again. So I DID NOT. I actually took the proverbial butcher knife to my schedule and cut out ANY unessential commitments. It was a scary but, in the end, very freeing thing. It took me a while to not feel guilty about it. But the real wake-up call for me was when my therapist said, "Do you really think you are so important that things cannot go on without you?"

The MS class was over and I felt like I did not need that kind of support any longer. I do see the importance of support groups, especially when you are in the middle of an "active" illness. But for me, it started to feel like a constant reminder of something I wanted to forget. It was not that I didn't want to face the disease, but I wanted to look into the future and wanted that outlook to be untainted. So I started working on future visioning. With the help of a friend and hypnotherapist, I first dealt with the anger and disappointment I felt with God and with MS, and then I started to create a future vision.

Now, ten years later, I still do the same thing. Every time I wake up in the morning I see myself as an older, wiser self, a grandma with short grey hair running on the beach and playing with a dog and some young grandchildren. I picture myself deeply involved in art and other activities I love—canoeing, hiking, doing yoga, laughing with friends, and walking hand in hand with my husband. I realized through this process that I had been kind of holding my breath for the few months directly following the diagnosis. I was afraid of my future. After doing this work, I felt much better and stronger and back in control.

For several years, things were stable and I was very active. I worked out several times a week and did pretty much the same things I had always done—though I had learned to be more "selfish" and to say NO. Then, all of a sudden, about five years ago my yearly MRI showed some new lesions. My neurosurgeon could hardly believe I didn't have any symptoms. She immediately put me on Betaseron and interferon injections every other day. I, of course, just trusted my doctor, scared out of my wits that I was going to get very ill. I continued my workouts and regular activities, but realized that the doctor's findings were a wake-up call. "Don't get too comfortable here!" I told myself.

Through one of my trainers at the gym I heard about a qigong practitioner who had made a big difference in her life. I went to see him, and he gave me exercises to do. I felt better right away. It wasn't that I didn't already feel good, because I did, but it was on a deeper level. I felt I was taking responsibility for myself and not just depending on medication. I continued to work with the qigong practitioner for over six months and felt very strong from the exercises. These exercises are a little different from the traditional qigong, as they were developed so that people who are paralyzed can do them. If all you can do is do the exercises in your mind, that's what you do. I've tried it and found that afterwards I feel completely charged and energetic.

At this point, I felt that there was still more that I could do for myself. I met an incredible hypnotherapist who encouraged me to get more involved with meditation. I started to meditate on a more regular basis and did a particular healing meditation. I also received some energy healing treatments, and it was brought to my attention that I might have some issues with candida. As so often happens in life, when you're on the right track things just fall into place. On my way home after the session I got a message from a friend saying, "This nutritionist I've been seeing is going to be on *Montel* this afternoon and they're going to be talking about MS. . . . Watch it." I missed the show, but was interested enough to look up "this nutritionist."

As soon as I saw Ann's website, I knew I wanted to read her book and go see her. It has now been about four years since I first saw Ann. Everything I learned from her made sense. I did have some candida and needed to clean my body out. Within the first two months of clearing my body of candida and following the diet and supplement protocol, I felt like a new woman. I felt like I had stepped out of a fog. I felt clear, clean, strong, and healthy. Qigong had been an almost daily part of my taking care of myself, and now I made a commitment to include yoga and felt my balance and strength improving.

I started getting a nagging feeling that the drugs I was still taking were not the answer, but the fear of a future with a disability stopped me from going off them. Then I started hearing stories of people living with MS without medication and people who were on medication and were not doing well. I thought about not being on medication, not having to take the detested injections, and not getting horrible bruises all over my stomach, thighs, and arms—not, not, not! When I talked to Ann about it, she assured me that I would know if and when I was ready to go off them. I talked to my neurologist and she was not very supportive, but agreed that it was up to me. Just at this point I got some blood work back, and it pointed to my liver numbers being somewhat elevated. Whoa, Silver! Warning lights!

Once again I had one of those "falling into place" experiences. When I went to the pharmacy to pick up my medication, it wasn't there. No problem, since I had a week before I was totally out. I called the doctor to make sure all the prescriptions and renewals were in order, went back to the pharmacy, and still no medicine. I was outraged that the pharmacy didn't contact the doctor when they realized they needed a renewal for the prescription, and that the doctor's office didn't respond soon enough to the delayed phone call from the pharmacy. I went to the pharmacy three times only to find out each time that, oops, they didn't have it. On and on this went, like a really bad Oliver and Hardy farce.

As this comedic tragedy was playing out around me, I went through every human emotion regarding the pharmaceutical theme, and it became clearer to me that I didn't need this medication. When I finally got the message from the pharmacy that the medication was ready for pick-up, I just erased it, called Ann and said, "I think I'm ready to do this!" Though it was not an easy decision, after examining my life, my emotions, talking to God, meditating, and releasing some anger, it felt like the right thing to do.

OUTCOME: It has now been one year and four months since I stopped the interferon injections. The MS symptoms that

I had had for years—numb toes and fingers, dizziness, and double vision—are pretty much totally gone, and I feel energetic, healthy and whole. I still meditate, do qigong and yoga, examine my life, visualize my future, and set intentions. I am present in my life and never ever take anything for granted. And, yes, I am very, VERY grateful.

SARITA

BACKGROUND: chicken pox; mononucleosis at age 18; very high stress with trauma history; sugar addict; severe asthma; allergy shots for ten years; one incident in the 1980s of waking up to a completely numb left arm, which did not resolve for one week

SYMPTOMS UPON VISIT: weakness and incoordination on left side, numb left foot, numb and spastic left hand, numbness in right hand, balance issues, foot drop on left side, walking difficulty with use of cane in winter and in unfamiliar places, mild to moderate fatigue

PHARMACEUTICALS TAKEN FOR MS: none

ANTIBIOTICS: My teeth showed signs of antibiotic use in my childhood, but memories of this are hazy.

DATE OF FIRST VISIT WITH ANN: January 2012

I graduated with my PhD in counseling psychology in 1988. Almost immediately afterwards, all the things I had stuffed emotionally started to emerge. I began psychotherapy in 1989, and it became apparent that I had buried memories of childhood trauma. I decided to discuss what I was discovering with my parents in January of 1991. Only later did I uncover the memory that I had been threatened not to tell my mother about my abuse or it would kill her. In my child heart, I had decided that I would be responsible for killing my mother if I talked. I had just talked.

My neurological symptoms began then. By April, my hands were so numb that I could not hold a fork or write without an orthotic. I had a sensation of tight bands around my chest, my eyesight was somewhat blurry, and I dragged my left foot when I walked. The worst part was my fatigue level. I was so exhausted daily that I could sleep twelve hours and wake up feeling as if I hadn't rested. I sometimes had a sensation of being pulled down when I was standing, which resulted in my not being able to stand for long periods of time. This was all terrifying.

I went in for an exam by my internist, who ordered an MRI. The group of doctors who looked at my scan as it emerged on screens that only they could see gave me no indication of what they saw. I was discharged to my internist, who told me that I had been diagnosed with MS. It is hard to explain what happens when you hear a diagnosis like that. For me, my first fear was that I would lose my eyesight and not be able to see my partner's eyes. Every step I took, I thought could be my last. I had no control over what my body was losing slowly, silently, and inexorably. It was terror as I had never known it.

Meanwhile, the very same month my mother was diagnosed with stage IV ovarian cancer. She was scheduled for a hysterectomy and I was supposed to go and be with her. I called her surgeon to say I did not know how or when to break the news of my MS diagnosis to her, as I did not want to jeopardize her recovery. I decided to call her after her surgery. She was so supportive despite her pain and status. That was all in April 1991. My mother died July 18, 1991. I could not feel her hands the last time I saw her alive. Deep in my unconscious I believed I had killed my mother. The connection between this and the emergence of my neurological symptoms was not lost on me.

I was referred to a neurologist, who gave me the usual exam. I went in with a list of things I thought I would need prescriptions for—a wheelchair, canes, and orthotics to help me write. He never asked me about precipitating stressors. He said he could put me in the hospital to get IV steroids to ease the current episode, and then gave me a book on MS and I was free to go home.

I was so confused. Now what? I read the book, which explained all the things that happen to people with MS: incontinence, loss of eyesight, loss of ability to walk, fatigue—you name it. All the worst-case scenarios were in there. I was horrified. I felt like all of that could happen to me at any minute.

I thought I should run to the hospital for help with steroids. But my partner said the words that changed my attitude about MS from then on: "If you really want to be sick, let them put you on IV steroids. If I were you, I would find an acupuncturist." I totally respected and trusted my partner, who is in the medical field, yet I could not see how acupuncture could help. Well, it really did help me. I started getting better and better.

Soon I decided that I did not really have MS and that my symptoms were all related to my trauma history. I continued my psychotherapy with an excellent therapist who helped me piece my childhood narrative back together. As I realized more about what had happened, my neurological symptoms continued to improve. I was on the road to recovery in the late 90s. Then around 2001 my walking began to become difficult. I was getting weaker on my left side and I had foot drop as well. Both hands had varying degrees of numbness, but not nearly as bad as in 1991. The emergence of these symptoms really scared me and began to shake me out of my denial about having MS.

I began having to plot out a course that included rest stops wherever I went. I could only grocery shop in a few aisles before my leg gave out, and I had to rest to restore it and then continue with the next few aisles. I was referred to a physical therapist and worked with her for three years. This helped me walk somewhat better, but I still had to carry groceries up the stairs where I lived one stair at a time. I'd put the bags down and pull myself up with the railing, and then grab the bags and do it all over again. There were sixteen stairs.

I decided I needed to find someone who could help me get stronger. I was referred to a wonderful personal trainer in 2008, and we began six months of orthopedic massage to get my muscles functional again and then did a weight-training program. I began to improve significantly and I was so hopeful. Then in spring 2009 I started to feel the characteristic symptoms of an MS exacerbation. I was exhausted and my left foot was numb. I decided to see the neurologist again and went in for my second MRI, nearly twenty years after my first one.

There I was again, in a skimpy patient's gown as a resident walked in and pulled up my MRI on the laptop. He was looking at my brain. I felt so powerless, even though he was very kind and professional. I asked him if I might have a benign case of MS, and he said it was possible, but that they didn't know enough about the disease. Then my neurologist walked in the door, and without even greeting me he said, "Do you have MS? Yes, you have MS!" He then proceeded to give me the same exam the resident had just administered. When an area of deficit was noted, he would look at the resident and say the part of my brain that was associated with the deficit. I am a psychologist and I know some neurophysiology, but he did not address me at all. When he finished, he said the MRI showed no new activity and that I was having a pseudo-exacerbation, a reactivation of old symptoms. He strongly advised me to get on the medications that were available. My other option was to see him annually to get repeat MRIs.

I had a curious response to this visit. Not only did I not shrink in terror; I got very angry at his disrespect. He never once asked me whether anything was going on with me psychologically. In fact, an incident had just occurred that triggered some of the very wounds present in my unconscious in 1991 when I was first diagnosed. I was determined never to see him again. So, without knowing it, he really helped me.

Five months later, my left knee gave out and I fell down a flight of sixteen stairs on my way out of the house to go to work. My denial about having MS was shattered. I knew I would have to move and got very serious about looking for ways to help myself. I had all of my amalgams removed to rid my body of the mercury toxicity they had caused. My thyroid crashed about then and I was exhausted, so I began to look at dietary options. My excellent physician suggested that I consider a food allergy elimination diet, which I did. When I slowly reintroduced food, I realized that I had a strong intolerance to gluten and yeast, so I discontinued both and felt much better. I read a book on a diet for MS that suggested cutting out dairy, soy, legumes, and perhaps eggs as well. I did this too and began to feel even better. I continued psychotherapy, and as my trauma was resolving, my body was also responding positively.

While researching thyroid conditions, I found some discussion of mycotoxins as an underlying cause of autoimmune diseases like MS. I asked my physician about this and she referred me to her nurse practitioner, who specialized in allergies and whose dad had MS. She recommended I get on the candida diet and gave me Ann Boroch's book, which I read. I REALLY balked at the idea of giving up sugar. I was astonished that my response was so strong after all I had already done. For me, sugar was energy and reward. I was addicted, and so I decided her program was too hard for me right then. The supplement regimen alone looked overwhelming. I was too tired. Besides, look at ALL I was already doing, I reasoned.

Yet I felt that a higher power had been leading me to every one of my great health-care team members so far, and I could not shake the notion that Ann Boroch was my next provider.

I emailed her and she responded right away. She is very orga-
nized, and though her program at first seemed too complex,
she quickly and deftly explained it to me.

I started Ann's diet eight months ago. I had already been
placed on Nystatin by my nurse practitioner, but did not get on
all of the supplements Ann recommends until five months ago.

Outcome: After eight months on Ann's program, strength is
returning to my left side, especially in my hip, and my grip
strength has improved. The first thing I noticed was that all the
numbness in my left foot went away, and it has not returned.
My energy level has not been this consistently good since I was
20!

My walking is also greatly improving This past summer
I attended a family wedding that was held on a mountain in
Montana, which would be a nightmare of a walking experience
for anyone with MS. I had to walk up a loose gravel road, over
an uneven lawn, and over a little foot bridge without handrails
to get to the ceremony, and had to negotiate uneven boardwalks
and a lawn at the reception location. Well, I did it, and I did
it well, with only a little help from my cane. I even danced. If
it wasn't for the improvement I had experienced on your program, I would not have even gone to this wedding!

My left arm is increasing in coordination. My trainer says
he notices steady improvements in my strength, and there is
full range of motion in my left ankle when he manipulates it,
which he could not do before. I am able to move my ankle and
foot on my own more and more, the spasticity is gone in my
left hand, and my foot drop is improving. I still have numbness
in my left fingers and use a cane in winter if it is icy or I am on
uneven ground. I am also noticing less effects from the heat
this summer. My vision has improved since my last visit to the
optometrist and is now 20/20.

I am so optimistic. I did not know MS could be improved, much less reversed. I am grateful to share my story if it helps somebody. To choose an alternative path to treat MS is scary. Like it says in Ann's book, every case of MS has layers, like an onion, that have to be peeled away. I had peeled away so many layers—I had completed twenty years of psychotherapy, resolved my thyroid issue, improved my strength, improved my diet, and I was not going to stop now because I couldn't give up sugar. I am determined to do what is in my power to do for my body. In fact, I see MS as a gift now. I never would have decided to care so well for my body without MS as a motivating force.

KIMBERLEE

BACKGROUND: fatigue and constipation since early 20s, high intake of coffee and sugar, numbness in right extremities, hair loss, red blotchy skin

SYMPTOMS UPON VISIT: fogginess, numbness from jaw to toes, tingling throughout body, extremely weak and constantly tired, spasticity in legs, loss of memory, blurred vision, balance issues and temporarily in wheelchair, extremely emotional for approximately one year

PHARMACEUTICALS TAKEN FOR MS: none

ANTIBIOTICS: As a small child I had cysts that had grown on both of my wrists, and each week the doctor repeatedly injected them with some type of pharmaceutical drug until they eventually dissipated. As a teen I was on an antibiotic for acne for approximately 6–8 months.

DATE OF FIRST VISIT WITH ANN: June 2011

While traveling abroad at age 25 my right leg went completely numb, which made it difficult to walk due to extreme stiffness and severe pain. I went to the doctor, who discounted my symptoms. After arriving back in the states, the symptoms completely disappeared, so I did not pursue any further action.

A couple of years later, I almost had a mysterious and dangerous fall in my home. After a few minutes I was feeling completely normal and so I continued on. A couple years after that, my right hand went completely numb and I lost use of it. It felt as if it were jammed in a permanent position. Upon visiting my doctor, I was sent for electrical stimulation therapy, which of course did nothing to help solve the problem except cause excruciating pain.

At age 40, my life completely changed. I took a mysterious fall at work and thought I just wasn't paying attention. A couple of days later while at home, my legs completely gave out and I fell backward onto an ottoman, landing on a wood tray and a stack of books. The next morning, I could hardly get out of bed, much less walk, so my sister took me to the doctor for x-rays and painkillers. It felt as if I had fractured my ribs and I could hardly move.

I went to see another doctor for more tests. While I was in the waiting room, my body completely gave up and I was unable to talk or walk. The nurse quickly rushed me in to see the doctor as tears streamed down my face. She just looked and me and sternly said, "What is wrong with you? Are you always this emotional?"

I was taken in for a CAT scan and later that week for an MRI, which confirmed that I did have MS. My neurologist wanted me to start medication that day, but I was very hesitant. He sent me home with a stack of literature regarding all of the current medications and told me to make sure to choose wisely because I was going to be on it for the rest of my life!

Luckily, a friend said to me, "If you change your diet, you change your life." At the same time, my best friend from Colorado sent me a text telling me about Ann and her book. By happenstance, I had just ordered the same book and it had arrived that day and was sitting next to me. I knew by now that I was receiving some type of divine guidance!

OUTCOME: I have been working with Ann for a little over a year and I am making great progress. I have completely changed my diet, and gave up my white mochas from Starbucks. I have only about 5 percent numbness, the wheelchair and walker are long gone, and my walking and balance have improved immensely, as well as my eyesight. I am now driving again, working part time, and slowly continuing to get back on track with my life.

After being on the program for eight months, I had another MRI, and all of my lesions except for one had completely shrunk. My neurologist was speechless, yet still insisting that I go on medication right away. That day I walked out of his office—and out of his life for good—with a HUGE smile! I'm feeling better and better as time passes. My skin looks almost flawless, and the best part about it is that total strangers walk up to me and ask me my secret. I just reply with much enthusiasm, "It's my diet!"

I plan to stick with Ann's diet as a total lifestyle change, and now I am studying nutrition and wellness, eager to regain my health completely and to help others in the future. I am eternally grateful to Ann for all of her help and could not imagine where I would be without her!

JIM

BACKGROUND: Sugar addiction since early childhood, standard American diet, and chronic earaches. Childhood: While riding my bike, I was frequently hit by cars that were pulling out of parking lots and driveways, and I "played" with insecticides and other chemicals. Teens: Drank lots of alcohol. Adulthood: Pulled a steel speaker tripod onto my head while passing out at an

Egyptian wedding (dented my forehead); was flipped from and pinned by a horse in the desert (no major injuries).

SYMPTOMS UPON VISIT: paresthesia below the waist, weakness, fatigue

PHARMACEUTICALS TAKEN FOR MS: none

ANTIBIOTICS: used antibiotics for childhood earaches; used them a few times in adulthood, but not excessively

DATE OF FIRST VISIT WITH ANN: November 2008

My first symptoms hit me when I was 29 years old, but I had no idea that they were related to a seemingly incurable disease that I would spend the rest of my life battling. I have been a musician all my life, though it wasn't until my early 20s that I decided to completely devote my life to learning, performing, and teaching music, resulting in a truly grand adventure.

In my mid to late twenties I was thoroughly immersed in studying Middle Eastern music at the University of Southern California, Santa Barbara, with a major in ethnomusicology. In my late twenties I had become a competent oud player (fretless lute), and my friends and I would often play at parties all through the night until dawn. After one such night during my twenty-eighth year, I awoke (late!) the next day to find my right hand, my picking hand, thick with pins and needles. Yes, I had played very hard the night before, probably overdoing it, I admitted to myself. As the tingling and numbness crept up my wrist and into my arm in the following days, I was convinced that I had damaged nerves in my neck or shoulder from playing too hard. I consulted massage therapists and researched stretching and posture techniques for musicians, such as the Alexander Technique. It seemed to be working, since the tingling fizzled away after a few months.

Right before my second research trip to Egypt (1999), the tingling came back; this time it eventually crept all the way to my bicep. I continued my physical therapy, but nothing seemed to affect it. However, this time random electric burst-attacks would overtake me. I think I looked like someone having a stroke, as the tingling would intensify to such an extreme degree that I would be forced to curl my arms inward, holding myself while bracing for the pain. These explosions were random and lasted a few minutes, but they were terrifying. I was sincerely scared and devastated that I was losing the ability to play music. I also remember dining with my fiancé and trying to use a fork and knife with a completely numb right arm and hand, dropping the knife repeatedly, and then breaking down in self-piteous tears.

In Egypt, I had to discuss this new handicap with my oud teacher, and he recommended playing qanun (ka-noon), a plucked zither, because the player sits with a straight back as opposed to the hunched-over position needed to play the oud. I was depressed and angry that I actually had to give up playing an instrument that I had devoted so many hours to, but also excited at the prospects of playing such a gorgeous and rare one (qanun). I have been a qanun player ever since.

After our first child was born in 2002, the symptoms hit me really hard. I woke up one morning with light tingling between my toes and in patches at the bottom of my feet. Of course, I thought it would disappear after a few minutes. After a few hours, it was still there and it seemed the tingling was spreading. Many of you know this story: After a few days the paresthesia had covered my feet and was traveling up my shins; in a few more days, it reached my knees and thighs; and eventually everything up to my waist was numb and tingling. I knew nothing about autoimmune diseases, so I figured it was a pinched nerve, or even a slipped disc. I saw a chiropractor; no result. I sought out massage and other physical therapies; no result. I even sought out an energy healer; no result.

The torturous experience of not being able to feel your feet, legs, and pelvis area, while simultaneously feeling heaviness or electric pulsing throughout, is indescribable. I had just welcomed my son into the world and was finishing my MA thesis, and now I was spiraling into depression and anxiety. We went to the emergency room in order to get a straight diagnosis. After some initial testing I was shocked to learn that a lumbar puncture, or spinal tap, would be necessary. They found pieces of myelin in my spinal fluid and suggested I see a neurologist.

Of course, after a visit to the neurologist I was diagnosed with MS. Earlier that day I left my house thinking that I was going to find out how to heal myself from a pinched nerve or slipped disc, and I came home with the darkest of clouds hanging over me and my family. The neurologist was smug and was already writing prescriptions for MS pharmaceuticals, essentially writing me off. I stormed out of there, determined to heal this my own way.

I researched everything I could find on MS, especially holistic and natural approaches. I found that Pepe & Hammond's *Reversing Multiple Sclerosis* as well as other sources were all agreeing in terms of a diet devoid of processed foods, grains, dairy, and sugars. I altered my diet accordingly, though still felt confused by the myriad therapies that "specialists" were espousing. My diet was cleaner than it had been, but some alternative sugars and starchy vegetables remained.

When I reflected back to 1999, I noticed a relapse pattern in which symptoms would strike every three years. However, I noticed that starting in 2005, the symptoms would increase at a yearly rate. The paresthesia would take my legs one year, a leg and a hip the next, and then the entire left hemisphere of my body. I began to recognize one of the relapse patterns I had read about. The relapses were occurring closer together and, in theory, they would never stop getting worse.

In 2008 I was driving home and Lisa Garr's *Aware Show* on KPFK (Los Angeles) was broadcasting on my car's radio. Being a musician, I don't usually listen to talk shows, but on this day I decided to listen. Ann Boroch was on the show and I was deeply affected not only by her story but by her passionate clarity regarding the root causes of MS and the methods that could be used in a holistic healing process. I bought her book and, again, modified my diet (which was already close to the candida diet). I felt reinvigorated in my battle.

That same year, I was hit with paresthesia on the entire left side of my body, intense lethargy, and depression. It was time to finally call Ann. After meeting with her I realized that I was missing one of the most important components towards rebuilding my nervous system: supplements. Of course, I was taking some, but nothing compared to the detailed and individualized regime that Ann prescribes. Because I was already on the candida diet, the addition of a new regime of supplements caused my symptoms to disintegrate in less than a month. The next relapse occurred a year or so later, and the symptoms disappeared in two to three weeks. The one after that was gone in two weeks. Now, this pattern was truly inspiring!

OUTCOME: In the last few years, when relapsing has occurred it has consisted of light tingling in my toes or what I call "phantom patches" of heat or electric pain on random body parts. I am energetic, physically active, and people comment on how much I seem to "glow." The diet and the supplement regime are crucial towards the healing process, but you must visualize, believe, know, and imagine that your body is healing and that you're steadfastly moving towards regeneration. And you will. I am grateful for Ann, and all the earlier sources, who helped guide me to the path of true healing.

JESSICA

BACKGROUND: chicken pox, frequent sinus infections, frequent stomach problems

SYMPTOMS UPON VISIT: numbness and tingling in arms and legs, crave sweets, bloating and gas, fatigue, anxiety, depression, memory loss, blurred vision, headaches, very high stress, worried constantly

PHARMACEUTICALS TAKEN FOR MS: none

ANTIBIOTICS: a lot

DATE OF FIRST VISIT WITH ANN: November 2010

I started working at the age of 13 and started holding high-stress positions at the age of 17, when I was an executive assistant. I have a history of stomach pains and had frequent sinus infections as well. After an endoscopy, colonoscopy, CT scan, and an IVP test, I was told I had an ulcer. I did the four-week treatment of three to four different medications that the doctor advised. I kept getting sinus infections well into my twenties, and eventually the doctor ordered a CT scan and they found I had a deviated septum. I had surgery for this at the age of 23.

While dealing with these health issues, I was also going to school part time and working forty hours or more a week. I would throw myself into work because I didn't want to face the reality of the abusive relationship I had been in for four years off and on with someone who cheated on me continuously. I couldn't get out of it because I really didn't know how to. Finally he left for a third time and I didn't run back. Instead I got into another relationship that was not abusive, but was full of neglect. During this time, I was full of emotions and was a binge drinker, and I would burst out and create emotional scenes.

Guilt and regret lay heavy after these situations. This relationship ended after two years because he was unfaithful.

In July 2009, I had a headache that lasted over a month. I was 24 years old then. My primary care physician ordered an MRI and referred me to a neurosurgeon, thinking I had temporal arthritis. The neurosurgeon said my MRI came back suspicious for MS and a mild form of Arnold Chiari malformation type I, and that there was no way I could have temporal arthritis because of my age. He advised I call my PCP about seeing a neurologist.

The neurologist concentrated more on the suspicion of MS than the headache issue. He said I had five to six lesions that showed demyelinating disease and asked if I had any numbness, tingling, or loss of vision or double vision. I told him the only thing I was experiencing were some vision problems due to the headaches, but nothing severe. I had a spinal tap done that also came back suspicious for MS. However, I still had no physical signs of MS other than the headache.

I didn't even know what MS was! He could not diagnose me, so he suggested another MRI six to eight months later. In May 2010 I had the second MRI, which showed twice as many lesions and that the previous lesions had gotten bigger and had active inflammation. When he asked if I had any physical symptoms or if I was feeling weak or tired, I said no and that I actually had started running on a treadmill about two to three times a week and felt fine, though I wasn't able to lose weight. He then referred me to get a second opinion.

The appointment I had with the second neurologist was in September 2010, and it did not go so well. She told me I would "eventually" have MS and I needed to start Rebif as soon as possible. I asked her how long I needed to take Rebif and she said for the rest of my life. I chuckled and looked at my now husband, who had come with me, and rolled my eyes. She then said, "Oh, you're one of those." The conversation got a little heated and I left with a hunger to know what this disease was all about. I was not going to take injections every day for the rest of my life because someone told me I would "eventually" have the disease. If I could prevent it in a healthier manner and not with injections, I was going to find a way.

I went to our local video and book store, and there was only one book on MS. That is where I came to find Ann Boroch's book. I was eager to learn about this disease and I was much stressed not knowing what options I had. My personality was already high stress, so to have added stress about my health made things worse for me. I contacted Ann after reading her patients' stories, and my husband and I decided to fly out to Los Angeles to meet with her. My appointment was almost two months out because of timing constraints for me. During this time I experienced tingling in my right arm. Since I hadn't met with Ann yet, I wasn't aware of what to do for this situation and was advised by the neurologist who had given me the second opinion to take prednisone, which I did, because I thought that "eventually" might become a reality.

When I finally met with Ann in November 2010, she was able to steer me in the right direction toward creating a healthy environment for my body to start to heal. I followed her path faithfully and felt better than I ever had! In January 2011, I went to a new neurologist because I felt I needed to have a neurologist watch over my progress. He ended up diagnosing me with MS due to the tingling I had experienced prior to seeing Ann and based on the results of my two MRIs and spinal tap. He ordered another MRI for six months out and advised I start Avonex. I told him I was going to take the natural route and had been working with Ann for a couple of months. He said, "If you were my wife or daughter, I would advise you to take the interferons." I said, "Thanks, but no thanks. I am going the natural route because I have done my own research on the interferons and have decided the natural route is best for me." He said that was fine, but we would still need to do the MRI in six months.

On March 11, 2011, it was my birthday. I thought I deserved to have a lot of fun the whole month, and the only way I knew to have fun back then was with alcohol and desserts. I started to drink again and satisfied my cravings for sweets. A few weeks into going back to my old habits, I ended up with my right arm going numb. I contacted Ann to let her know. I felt so bad because I didn't want to disappoint her and was worried about what she was going to say when I asked for her guidance. She said, "It's okay if you have fallen off course. You will find your way and realize what is more important."

The numbness went away soon after getting back on Ann's plan and I thought to myself, "WOW, this really works!" When I saw the neurologist a couple months later to order the third MRI, he questioned me about the exacerbation spontaneously going away without steroids. I laughed and said I was a true believer that the natural route really worked. The result from the third MRI showed I had one new lesion with active inflammation. The neurologist called me on a Saturday to tell me and advised that I start the interferons. I declined once again because even though there was one new lesion with active inflammation, it was by far better than having a dozen more new lesions with active inflammation, which might have been expected based on the MRI I had the year before. For me that meant the path I was following with Ann was working.

Outcome: I have since taken a lower stress job and finally received an associate's degree in business administration. I have seen a hypnotherapist to help me clear up the emotional pain I endured in the past, and I have never felt better mentally or physically. I learned that nobody was going to watch what I ate and I had to hold myself accountable so that I wouldn't experience an exacerbation like the one I had back in April 2011. Since then, I have not had another exacerbation. My husband and I found out we were pregnant in January 2012, and we are expecting a little boy in September 2012. Although I have had my challenges with certain cravings, I know that what I eat will not only affect me but will affect him as well. I know where I want to be and that is to continue to be symptom-free after the baby is born and thereafter, to keep up the lifestyle changes that Ann has provided, and to teach others that they too are in control of healing their own body.

KERRY

BACKGROUND: chicken pox, mononucleosis at age 16, shingles, frequent migraine headaches from age 16 to 30, high periods of stress during career, numerous cases of strep throat treated with antibiotics, high sugar and carbohydrate cravings

SYMPTOMS UPON VISIT: cold hands and feet, numbness and tingling, sweet and carbohydrate cravings, bloating, anxiety, high stress, headaches, insomnia, double vision, poor memory and concentration, mood swings, dizziness, gait difficulties

PHARMACEUTICALS TAKEN FOR MS: steroids, Rebif (4 months, bad reaction), Copaxone (8 months)

ANTIBIOTICS: 25 rounds in lifetime (approx.)

DATE OF FIRST VISIT WITH ANN: August 2011

I will always remember the beginning of my MS journey at the age of 47 years old. It was a late afternoon when I walked into a colleague's office for a meeting, sat down and noticed the words on a document I was reading were a bit blurry. I excused myself and went to get my saline solution, thinking my contact lenses were dry. Saline did not help. Since it was the end of the day, I left my office and drove home.

Once I reached home, I immediately took out my contacts and put my glasses on, thinking I just had an irregular pair of lenses. No such luck. The blurred vision remained and I made a mental note to call my eye doctor first thing in the morning. The next morning after getting ready for work, I sat on the couch looking for my doctor's phone number, when all of a sudden my right arm and right side of my face went completely numb. I immediately thought, "I'm having a stroke." I calmly went upstairs to wake my daughter to tell her I needed to be seen in the ER.

After a myriad of tests, including a CAT scan, MRI, EKG, and blood and spinal tests, the head ER doctors told me I had MS and asked if I knew what that meant. I had six total lesions on both sides of the brain, and it was evident the disease was active at the time of the MRI. I remained very calm, because four years earlier I had spent quite a bit of time emotionally reacting to my younger brother's diagnosis of MS. I was not shocked. Instead, I was immediately hopeful because he had been working with Ann and was miraculously ridding himself of his MS symptoms as a result of her program.

I was admitted to the hospital for three days of IV steroids to help relieve the inflammation. I met with my neurologist the following week, and she called my episode a CIS—clinically isolated syndrome—with probable MS. My eyesight three weeks later was at 90 percent and still improving, but anxiety attacks were increasing. A second MRI was performed on my neck and spine and showed no lesions present. I started the drug Rebif, an interferon used for the relapsing-remitting form of MS. The side effects were unpleasant, as I always had flu-like symptoms and constant headaches.

Two months after my diagnosis, my brother took me to Los

Angeles to meet Ann. I had already read both of her books and was so anxious to start the 90-day program and beat this disease. I REALLY believed that I could get rid of the MS symptoms by changing the way I ate and my lifestyle in general. I started the nutrition and supplement program, and I can truly say that I have never been so serious about anything in my life. "I may have MS, but it does not have me" were words I'd repeat on a daily basis. Soon my energy level was coming back and I was feeling so much better. I was thinking positively and was very confident about my recovery. I have my brother to thank for leading me to Ann.

Over the next few months I religiously met with Ann via Skype sessions, during which she altered my supplements to meet my progression. I had a blood test two months after starting the Rebif therapy and my liver was showing signs of damage. I had two more blood tests and my liver enzymes were up four times the normal rate. I immediately checked in with Ann, and she again adjusted my supplements to compensate for the weakness of my liver. Needless to say, Ann had me continue the 90-day program and I did not waiver. She always said, "The body has an amazing ability to heal."

I explained to my neurologist that I was on a rigorous diet and supplement program, that my brother who was diagnosed with the same type of MS was having complete success with this program, and that his MRIs after four years were showing great improvement such that lesions were shrinking and even disappearing. So I chose to start a new drug therapy, the one my brother was on, which is Copaxone. I wanted to give this drug a try and scheduled my next MRI for June 2012, one year after my diagnosis and six months after starting Copaxone.

OUTCOME: It has been fourteen months since my diagnosis and I've never felt better. I am following Ann's recommended diet 90 percent of the time and continue taking her suggested daily supplements. I lead a less stressful life and have come to realize how the food that I eat has a direct effect on how I feel each day. In fact, my second MRI stated, "Overall improvement in number, size, and enhancement of the bihemispheric T2 hyperintensities compatible demyelination." My neurologist said she had to read the results a few times, as my results were not commonplace with this mysterious disease. Although she could not specify the exact reason for the dramatic improvement in my MRI, she said I was responding to treatment and advised me to continue what I was doing, which is a combination of Copaxone and the strict diet and supplement program that Ann is monitoring.

I am so very grateful to Ann for sharing her personal story and for all her research and putting her program into print. I find myself telling anyone with an ailment how the power of diet and a nutritional makeover can provide results far beyond their belief.

LEANNE

BACKGROUND: chicken pox, frequent ear infections and colds, mononucleosis at age 15, high periods of stress, high sugar intake

SYMPTOMS UPON VISIT: cold hands and feet, numbness and tingling, hypoglycemia, crave sweets, itchy skin and feet, bloating and gas, anxiety, frequent thirst, depression

PHARMACEUTICALS TAKEN FOR MS: Avonex and steroids

ANTIBIOTICS: 60 rounds in lifetime

DATE OF FIRST VISIT WITH ANN: March 2001

I went to college in Boston, about ninety miles from where I grew up, and majored in music and business management.

After graduating, I moved to Los Angeles, where I got a dream job working for Virgin Records in the art department. It was a high-stress, fast-paced world of work and parties, and parties and work.

All that changed in January, when my legs started to go numb. My doctor told me that I had a pinched nerve and put me on anti-inflammatory drugs. When I called a week later to tell her that the numbness hadn't subsided, she said I was over-reacting and needed to give it more time. I did exactly that and gave it another week.

On Super Bowl Sunday that year, my right arm and the right side of my face went numb. That was when my doctor decided I needed to come in for some tests. She sent me to a neurologist for a nerve conduction study. It came back normal. I started to panic. It was frustrating not to have anyone in the medical field at least acknowledge that something was going on with my body. It couldn't have all been in my head!

Then my eyesight went when I was driving to work one day. My assistant had to come and pick me up. She took me back to my doctor, and I finally went in for a CAT scan. When the results came in, the neurologist sat me down and told me I had MS: "You'll have it for the rest of your life. The best thing for you to do is start the medication immediately." Wow—that was a heavy thing to be told when just a month ago I'd been a healthy 25-year-old. I immediately started a steroid drip every day. A nurse came to my house and hooked me up to the drip. I lost about ten pounds (and I've always had a problem keeping weight on), and I couldn't sleep, but I also couldn't sit at work for eight hours. My body was a mess.

Fortunately, someone in my office said they used to work with a woman who had had MS and who was now working with people who were suffering from many different diseases. That person was Ann. I called her and she got me in to see her within two days. I spent an hour and a half with her, and that was when I finally found someone who helped me understand my disease and inspired me to want to beat it. I've never been a person who takes the easy road, and this one wasn't easy. I had a lot of emotional issues that needed to be dealt with. My diet was horrible, and I was a physical ball of stress! Fortunately, about three or four months earlier, after having had a definite drinking problem, I quit drinking.

It also wasn't easy convincing my family that the treatment plan Ann was recommending was the right thing for me to do. I now live about three thousand miles away from home, so the call to my mother telling her that I was going to stop treatment and go the holistic route wasn't an easy one. Luckily for me, my family has always been open-minded about things once they know I've thought them through.

After stopping the steroid treatments and without starting the medication, I took Ann's nutrition and supplement suggestions and put them to work. My energy level came back, and then some, and I started to feel like my healthy self again. The feeling slowly returned to my body. My balance came back and my eyesight returned to normal. I also started to feel confident that I had made the correct decision. Just by changing my diet and noticing what was going on with my body more, I came to realize that I could heal myself from this disease. I also started working with Ann on emotional situations that we felt were hindering my healing. After some work—and yes, it was a lot of work—I was able to start letting go of emotional baggage that I had been carrying around for years. I had a lot of insecurities and fear that added to dealing with this dreaded disease.

I had lived my life trying to please everyone, and being diagnosed with MS was my wake-up call that it was time to take care of me. Ann was instrumental in teaching me how to do this, and she was also a fantastic support system when I had lapses. With Ann, it was never, "You have to do this." It was always, "When your time is right you'll see that this is what you need to do." And she couldn't have made me more comfortable during my growing pains. At her suggestion, I also started doing yoga, and I'm now working on my third teacher's certification. I wanted to start working with other people who have MS. Ann has given me so much, and the least I can do is pass on the knowledge and support that she has given me throughout the years.

OUTCOME: I have been symptom-free for almost twelve years and have had no further attacks. Currently, I am not taking any pharmaceutical medications for MS. I now live in Northern California and still work in the music industry. The job is stressful, but I keep Ann's lessons with me every day and take any lull in energy as a sign to chill out. I am still doing yoga, but unfortunately not teaching (yet) up north.

I got married and had my first child on October 4, 2011. So to say the past eight years have been stress-free couldn't be farther from the truth. Yet I had no attacks when planning the wedding or during my pregnancy, and Kelly is a healthy boy. I didn't have any issues with fatigue or even huge hormonal peaks during my pregnancy or when I was breastfeeding Kelly for his first nine months. I was able to go back to work six weeks after his birth. I would get tired every now and again, but who is to say that that is from MS and not the normal reaction to a new mother's lack of sleep.

I also keep the lessons that Ann has taught me in mind when raising Kelly. I am not fearful when asking his doctors questions to make sure that my husband and I are well educated about all vaccinations and medications before making any decisions. Working with Ann gave me the power I needed in order to question medical professionals and not just trust them out of fear.

DINAH

BACKGROUND: childhood chicken pox, a lot of stomach issues, mercury fillings, high stress

SYMPTOMS UPON VISIT: hospitalized with optic neuritis and severe headache

PHARMACEUTICALS TAKEN FOR MS: Rebif, Neurontin, 3 rounds of steroids, Xanax

ANTIBIOTICS: 27 rounds

DATE OF FIRST VISIT WITH ANN: July 2010

In February 2010, I received a diagnosis of probable MS during an emergency room visit. I had gone to the ER for blurred vision and severe headaches. The emergency room doctor thought it was probably MS upon initial treatment and had me checked into the hospital. This came as a complete shock. I was 47 and thought I was too old for MS.

Within weeks of the first hospital visit, I lost sight in one eye from the optic neuritis and had to start walking with a cane due to muscle weakness in my left leg. I experienced vertigo so badly that friends had to drive me to work for two weeks. As the days and months went by, I also experienced bowel and kidney dysfunction, burning all over my body, loss of strength, fatigue, tingling in my feet and legs, electric shock sensations when I bent my head forward, and depression. I had always enjoyed an active lifestyle, which included hiking, running, biking, and outdoor events. I was scared and depressed by all these changes to my body.

I started taking Rebif and Neurontin, but my symptoms continued to worsen. I continued to lose strength in my legs and whole body. I kept going to work, but had to walk with a cane. The fatigue was so bad I had to take naps at lunch on a mat on the floor in my office. I could no longer run, walk very far, or bike. I felt like my quality of life was over. I did not want to live like this and started contemplating my exit strategy.

Then a friend mentioned a book entitled *Healing Multiple Sclerosis* by Ann Boroch. I got the book and decided to contact Ann. She outlined the program she had used to heal her body of MS, and I started the program on July 1, 2010. I put all my prescription medication in the garbage and spent one week in bed while my body detoxed all the chemicals I had been given over the last few months.

During the detox phase, there were times I felt I was not going to make it, nor did I really want to go on. Then day by day, with strict adherence to the program, I began to recover my strength and energy. I started very slowly. I walked around my neighborhood, and by the time I got home I was very tired. Then, slowly, the walks became longer—from ten-minutes to fifteen minutes to thirty and eventually an hour. By this time I was able to hike again.

I joined a gym and began to exercise five to six times per week. I started by lifting five to ten pounds of weight on the weight machines twice a week. In addition to building strength in my upper body, I began to slowly rebuild the muscles in my legs using the StairMaster and elliptical machine. Some days I did not know how I would even find enough energy to walk into the building and then walk to the exercise equipment, but I did. Soon I could run and bike again. I started running one-half mile at 4.5 miles per hour, and increased the distance each week by four-tenths of a mile and the speed by .2 miles per hour. Slowly I started building up mileage on the bike, starting at three miles.

Over the last two years, I completed two triathlons and numerous 5ks. I even have a few medals from these events. To me, the medals represent the importance of strength and courage. Never give up no matter what life may have in store for you. Just keep believing in yourself and know that if you put one foot in front of the other, you will cross the finish line and make your goal.

Even though I was angry that I had MS, I did not give up my faith in God. I continued to affirm healing of my body and soul. I am very blessed and grateful for the healing I have experienced.

OUTCOME: As a result of being on the program, I am now almost completely symptom-free. My eyesight continues to recover even though the ophthalmologist stated it would not. I continue to know and believe it will fully recover. Thanks to following the diet and supplement plan outlined in Ann's book, I have my life back. I am active, enjoy each day, and love life again. It is not always easy to follow the diet since I have to prepare almost everything I eat, but that is a lot easier than losing my quality of life.

It is very important to meditate, exercise, and affirm good health on a daily basis. Faith, belief and commitment will get you 80 percent of the way, and the rest will be easy. Today I am able to work out five times a week, work full time at my current job, and enjoy life to the fullest.

CHAPTER SEVENTEEN

CONCLUSION

A CURE IS POSSIBLE

Why does it sound so unreasonable to talk about a "cure" for MS? Maybe because we've been brainwashed by the medical establishment to believe it's not possible. The belief that it's incurable is only valid if you own it.

The *Merriam-Webster's Collegiate Dictionary* defines *cure* as "recovery or relief from a disease" and "a complete or permanent solution or remedy." One of the definitions from the *Oxford English Dictionary* is "restoration to health." Cures do occur in individuals. I'm one of them. There are cures for MS, cancer, and even AIDS, but we just don't hear about them because cures would put the pharmaceutical companies out of business. In our country today, despite all our technology and education, greed is a higher priority than health. That's why we're one of the sickest nations in the world—thirty-seventh on the world health index, to be exact.

When it comes to getting well, you have many approaches and methods to choose from. There is no right or wrong way to get to the light at the end of the tunnel. Some people use only alternative methods to get well; some use a combination of Western and alternative approaches. You do not have to ignore or divorce Western medicine. Explore all options, become educated, be open, and trust what you feel is best for you.

A cure for MS, or any chronic disease, does not come in one pill or one herb, nor does it happen overnight. It requires a combination of protocols that turn the body and mind around. Removing inflammation and infection for a long enough period of time is the key to remission and reversal. To do that, the most important step is to bring candida back into balance in the body, which also puts viruses into dormancy and rids the body of parasites and unhealthy bacteria.

The first goal in beating MS is stopping the progression, the second is experiencing a reversal of symptoms, and the third is having a permanent remission, which means being asymptomatic even during periods of stress. Those who are at a more progressed stage of MS might only accomplish stopping the progression. That needs to be seen as a big win. Others will reverse the symptoms and go into remission. The signifying factor will not necessarily be an MRI free of lesions. Lesions may decrease, go away completely, or show up but stay inactive for the rest of your life. Your progress is determined by how you feel—now, one year from now, five years from now, and twenty to thirty years from now.

THE WINNING SECRET

The secret to changing the cellular function of your body lies in what you believe. Those beliefs send messages to your central nervous system, which dictate every process in your body. So first make the choice to be healthy. Then claim that belief with conviction each day, and live it through your every thought, feeling, and action. With time, diligence, and patience, your body will mirror that belief.

PART FOUR

~~~~~

YOUR TREATMENT PLAN

CANDIDA HEALTH QUESTIONNAIRE

This questionnaire will help you and your health-care practitioner evaluate how *Candida albicans* may be linked to your health problems, but it won't provide a definitive yes or no answer as to whether you have candidiasis. A comprehensive history and physical examination are an important part of the evaluation, and laboratory studies and other types of tests may also be appropriate.

The questionnaire, developed by William G. Crook, MD, lists factors in your medical history that promote the growth of *Candida albicans* (Section A), as well as symptoms commonly found in individuals with yeast-connected illness (Sections B and C).

For each "yes" answer in Section A, circle the point score next to the question. Total your score, and record it at the end of the section. Then move on to Sections B and C, and score as directed. At the end of the questionnaire, you will add your scores to get your grand total.

SECTION A: History   **Point Score**

1. Have you taken any tetracyclines (Sumycin, Panmycin, Vibramycin, Minocin, etc.) or other antibiotics for acne for one month (or longer)?   50
2. Have you at any time in your life taken other "broad spectrum" antibiotics for respiratory, urinary, or other infections for two months or longer? Or for shorter periods four or more times in a one-year span?   50
3. Have you ever taken an antibiotic drug—even one round/course?   6
4. Have you at any time in your life been bothered by persistent prostatitis, vaginitis, or other problems affecting your reproductive organs?   25
5. Have you been pregnant two or more times?   5
   One time?   3
6. Have you taken birth control pills for more than two years?   15
   For six months to two years?   8
7. Have you taken prednisone, Decadron, or other cortisone-type drugs by mouth or inhalation for more than two weeks?* 15
   For two weeks or less?   6
8. Does exposure to perfumes, insecticides, fabric shop odors, or other chemicals provoke moderate to severe symptoms?   20
   Mild symptoms?   5
9. Are your symptoms worse on damp, muggy days or in moldy places?   20

*The use of nasal or bronchial sprays containing cortisone and/or other steroids promotes yeast overgrowth in the respiratory tract.

247

10. Have you had athlete's foot, ringworm, "jock itch" or
    other chronic fungus infections of the skin or nails?
    Have such infections been severe or persistent?   20
          Mild to moderate?   10
11. Do you crave sugar?   10
12. Do you crave breads?   10
13. Do you crave alcoholic beverages?   10
14. Does tobacco smoke really bother you?   10

Total Score Section A   _____

SECTION B: Major Symptoms

For each symptom you experience, enter the appropriate number in the
point score column:

> If a symptom is occasional or mild: score 3 points
> If a symptom is frequent and/or moderately severe: score 6 points
> If a symptom is severe and/or disabling: score 9 points

Total the score and record it at the end of this section.

                                                          Point Score

1. Fatigue or lethargy   _____
2. Feeling "drained"   _____
3. Poor memory   _____
4. Feeling "spacey" or "unreal"   _____
5. Inability to make decisions   _____
6. Numbness, burning, or tingling   _____
7. Insomnia   _____
8. Muscle aches   _____
9. Muscle weakness or paralysis   _____
10. Pain and/or swelling in joints   _____
11. Abdominal pain   _____
12. Constipation   _____
13. Diarrhea   _____
14. Bloating, belching, or intestinal gas   _____
15. Troublesome vaginal burning, itching, or discharge   _____
16. Prostatitis   _____
17. Impotence   _____
18. Loss of sexual desire or feeling   _____
19. Endometriosis or infertility   _____
20. Cramps and/or other menstrual irregularities   _____
21. Premenstrual tension   _____
22. Attacks of anxiety or crying   _____
23. Cold hands or feet and/or chilliness   _____
24. Shaking or irritability when hungry   _____

Total Score Section B   _____

SECTION C: Other Symptoms*

For each symptom you experience, enter the appropriate number in the point score column:

If a symptom is occasional or mild:	score 3 points
If a symptom is frequent and/or moderately severe:	score 6 points
If a symptom is severe and/or disabling:	score 9 points

Total the score and record it at the end of this section.

Point Score

1. Drowsiness _____
2. Irritability or jitteriness _____
3. Lack of coordination _____
4. Inability to concentrate _____
5. Frequent mood swings _____
6. Headaches _____
7. Dizziness and/or loss of balance _____
8. Pressure above ears or feeling of head swelling _____
9. Tendency to bruise easily _____
10. Chronic rashes or itching _____
11. Psoriasis or recurrent hives _____
12. Indigestion or heartburn _____
13. Food sensitivities or intolerances _____
14. Mucus in stools _____
15. Rectal itching _____
16. Dry mouth or throat _____
17. Rash or blisters in mouth _____
18. Bad breath _____
19. Foot, hair, or body odor not relieved by washing _____
20. Nasal congestion or postnasal drip _____
21. Nasal itching _____
22. Sore throat _____
23. Laryngitis or loss of voice _____
24. Cough or recurrent bronchitis _____
25. Pain or tightness in chest _____
26. Wheezing or shortness of breath _____
27. Urinary frequency, urgency, or incontinence _____
28. Burning on urination _____
29. Erratic vision or spots in front of eyes _____
30. Burning or tearing of eyes _____
31. Recurrent ear infections or fluid in ears _____
32. Ear pain or deafness _____

Total Score Section C _____
Total Score Section B _____
Total Score Section A _____
Grand Total Score (add totals from sections A, B, and C) _____

*Although the symptoms in this section occur commonly in clients with yeast-connected illness, they also occur commonly in clients who do not have candida.

The Grand Total Score will help you and your practitioner decide if your health problems are yeast-connected. Scores for women will run higher because seven items apply exclusively to women, while only two apply exclusively to men.

- Yeast-connected health problems are almost certainly present in women with scores over 180 and in men with scores over 140.

- Yeast-connected health problems are probably present in women with scores over 120 and in men with scores over 90.

- Yeast-connected health problems are possibly present in women with scores over 60 and in men with scores over 40.

- Scores of less than 60 for women and less than 40 for men indicate that yeast are less apt to cause health problems.

Source: This questionnaire is adapted from William G. Crook, MD, *The Yeast Connection Handbook* (Jackson, TN: Professional Books, Inc, 2000). Used with permission.

FOODS TO EAT

Now that you can better appreciate the nutritional needs of your body, it should be easier to stick to the candida-cure diet, knowing that it will both nourish you, eliminate candida, and help toward healing MS. The following lists give you general guidelines about the foods that are beneficial to eat and do not promote the growth of yeast, and the foods that you need to avoid because they *do* promote yeast overgrowth.

Be aware, however, that everyone's body chemistry is different. Some people have sensitivities or allergies to certain foods on the "Foods to Eat" list, so observe your body in case it reacts negatively to any of the foods. Symptoms such as fatigue, itching, rapid heart rate, gas, burping, bloating, constipation, diarrhea, and headaches are signs that you need to stay away from those particular foods. Listen to your body. It will tell you what it wants and does not want. Be aware, though, that when your body is toxic, you are going to crave more of the offending foods. But as you cleanse, your body will start to desire healthier foods, and it will be easier to trust the signals that it gives you.

Animal Protein (antibiotic- and hormone-free as much as possible; eat 2–4 ounces daily or no less than 3 times a week)

Beef, bison, lamb (grass-fed; no more than a 3- to 4-ounce serving once a week; most people with MS do best avoiding red meat entirely because it increases inflammation; prepare rare to medium-rare and eat with nonstarchy vegetables)
Chicken, turkey, and duck
Eggs
Fish (no shellfish for 3 months, then small amounts only)

NOTE: Due to ongoing ocean pollution from many sources, including nuclear leaks at the Fukushima Daiichi power plant in Japan, stay up to date on which fish become contaminated.

Grains (whole and unrefined only)

Amaranth

Breads (gluten-, yeast-, sugar-, and dairy-free)

Brown rice (short and long grain, brown basmati; limit to 2–3 times a week)

Brown rice cakes and crackers (limit to 2–3 times a week)

Buckwheat

Kañiwa

Millet

Oats (gluten-free,* only after 3 months on program)

Pasta (brown rice, buckwheat, and quinoa only; limit to 1 time a week)

Quinoa

Sorghum

Tapioca

Teff

Wild rice

Yucca

Vegetables

All (except corn, mushrooms, peas, and potatoes)

Sweet potatoes, yams, and winter squash (limit to 2–3 servings a week total)

NOTE: Limit or avoid nightshade-family vegetables for the first 3 months (eggplant, tomatoes, and peppers) because they can cause inflammation. If you eat them and your symptoms increase, avoid completely for the first 3 months and then reintroduce in small amounts if you wish.

Beans and Legumes

Avoid this group entirely for the first 3 months of the program because of their potential to cause inflammation and their high starch levels, which raise blood sugar. After this time period, you may eat beans and legumes in small amounts, except for

---

*Oats do not contain gluten; however, they are sometimes cross-contaminated with other gluten grains. Therefore, when eating oats, purchase a brand that ensures that it is gluten-free, such as Bob's Red Mill.

Dry mustard (or small amounts of mustard made with apple cider vinegar)

Fresh herbs (basil, parsley, etc.)

Kelp flakes (Bragg Organic Sea Kelp Delight Seasoning)

Mayonnaise (see Recipes)

Pepper

Rice vinegar (unseasoned and unsweetened only—store in refrigerator)

Sea salt

Spices (without sugar, MSG, or additives); favor ginger and turmeric (anti-inflammatory)

Beverages

Bragg Apple Cider Vinegar Drinks (Ginger Spice, Limeade, and Sweet Stevia only)

Herbal teas (red clover, peppermint, green, etc.)

Unsweetened almond, coconut, and hemp milk

Unsweetened mineral water (Gerolsteiner)

Water (filtered, purified, or distilled only)

Sweeteners

Chicory root (Just Like Sugar)

Lo han (luo han)

Stevia

Xylitol (small amounts; The Ultimate Sweetener)

Miscellaneous

Cacao powder (raw, unsweetened; small amounts after 3 months)

Carob (unsweetened; small amounts after 3 months because it is a legume)

Cocoa powder (unsweetened; small amounts after 3 months)

Coconut butter (organic)

Dill pickles (made without vinegar only; Bubbies)

Gums/mints (sweetened with lo han, stevia, or xylitol)

Salsa (without sugar or vinegar, except apple cider vinegar)

Sauerkraut (made without vinegar only; Bubbies)

FOODS TO AVOID

Avoid the foods on this list while you are on the candida-cure diet. After three months, you may include the foods below marked with an asterisk (*). Add one food at a time every third day and see if your body reacts—i.e., rapid heartbeat, itching, bloating and gas, constipation, fatigue, or worsening of your MS symptoms. If this happens, keep these foods out of your diet for another three months and then try again if you wish.

Animal Protein

Bacon (except turkey bacon without nitrates and hormones)

Hotdogs (except chicken and turkey hotdogs without nitrates and hormones)

Pork

Processed and packaged meats

Sausages (except chicken and turkey sausages that are gluten-, hormone-, antibiotic-, and nitrate-free)

Shellfish* (small amounts after 3 months)

Tuna (all: toro, albacore, ahi, etc., including canned)

Grains

Barley

Breads (except gluten-, dairy-, yeast-, and sugar-free, but not containing the grains listed here)

Cereals (except gluten-, dairy-, and sugar-free)

Corn (tortillas, polenta, popcorn, chips, etc.)

Crackers (except gluten-, dairy-, yeast-, and sugar-free; do not eat any with corn, potato, and/or white flour)

Kamut

Oats* (use gluten-free after 3 months)

Pasta (except brown rice, buckwheat, and quinoa)

Pastries

Rye

Spelt
Triticale
White flours
White rice
Wheat (refined)
Whole wheat

Vegetables

Corn
Mushrooms
Peas
Potatoes

Beans and Legumes

Avoid these entirely for the first 3 months of the program be-cause of their potential to cause inflammation and their high starch levels, which raise blood sugar. If you reintroduce, eat small amounts only once or twice a week, but continue to stay off soy (tofu, soybeans, tamari, and ponzu sauce) and fermented soy products (miso, tempeh, etc.).

Nuts and Seeds

Cashews*
Peanuts, peanut butter
Pistachios*

Oils

Canola oil
Corn oil
Cottonseed oil
Peanut oil
Processed oils and partially hydrogenated or hydrogenated oils
Soy oil

Dairy

Cheeses (all, including cottage and cream cheese)
Buttermilk
Cow's milk

Goat's milk and cheese (raw okay after 3 months, small amounts)
Ice cream
Kefir
Margarine
Sheep cheese (raw okay after 3 months, small amounts)
Sour cream
Yogurt

NOTE: Pregnant and nursing women should not eat raw dairy products.

Fruits

Apricots*
Bananas*
Cherries*
Cranberries* (unsweetened after 3 months)
Dried fruits (all, including apricots, dates, figs, raisins, cranberries, prunes, etc.)
Guavas*
Grapes*
Juices (all, sweetened or unsweetened)
Kiwis*
Mangoes*
Melons*
Nectarines*
Oranges*
Papayas*
Peaches*
Pears*
Pineapples*
Plums*
Persimmons*
Pomegranates*
Tangerines*

Beverages

Alcohol

Caffeinated teas (except green tea)
Coffee (caffeinated and decaffeinated)
Energy drinks (e.g., Red Bull, vitamin waters)
Fruit juices
Kefir
Kombucha
Sodas (diet and regular)
Rice and soy milks

Condiments

Gravy
Jams and jellies
Ketchup
Mayonnaise (see Recipes)
Mustard (unless made with apple cider vinegar; small amounts)
Pickles
Relish
Salad dressing (unless sugar-free and made with apple cider vinegar or unsweetened rice vinegar)
Sauces with vinegars and sugar
Soy sauce, ponzu, and tamari sauce
Spices that contain yeast, sugar, or additives
Vinegars (all, except raw, unfiltered apple cider vinegar and unsweetened rice vinegar—keep refrigerated)
Worcestershire sauce

Sweeteners

Agave nectar (Nectevia)
Artificial sweeteners, such as aspartame (Nutrasweet), acesulfame K, saccharin, and sucralose (Splenda)
Barley malt
Brown rice syrup
Brown sugar
Coconut sugar/nectar
Corn syrup
Dextrose

Erythritol (Nectresse, Swerve, Truvia)

Fructose, products sweetened with fruit juice

Honey (raw or processed; raw honey may be used medicinally)

Maltitol

Mannitol

Maltodextrin

Maple syrup

Molasses

Raw or evaporated cane juice crystals

Sorbitol

White sugar

Yacon syrup

Miscellaneous

Cacao/chocolate* (unless sweetened with stevia or xylitol; small amounts after 3 months)

Candy

Carob* (unsweetened, small amounts after 3 months because it is a legume)

Cookies

Donuts

Fast food and fried foods

Fruit strips

Gelatin

Gum (unless sweetened with stevia or xylitol)

Jerky (beef, turkey)

Lozenges/mints (unless sweetened with lo han, stevia, or xylitol)

Muffins

Pastries

Pizza

Processed food (TV dinners, etc.)

Smoked, dried, pickled, or cured foods

FIVE-WEEK
NUTRITIONAL MAKEOVER

Modifying your diet to get healthy can be a challenge. To be successful, it helps to understand that these dietary changes are not about deprivation—they are about eating foods that will help clear infection and inflammation, detoxify and rebuild your body, and restore health. If you slip up and eat something that's not on the plan, don't feel guilty. Just get back on track and keep going. When guilt gets in the way, you're more likely to continue eating foods that aren't good for you.

The following plan helps you to eliminate foods over a period of five weeks so that you can ease into the change in diet. However, you may jump right into the candida-cure diet and supplement protocol instead of doing the five-week nutritional makeover if you choose. The items with asterisks (*) may be reintroduced into your diet after three months.

Begin your supplement protocol after you complete the five-week nutritional makeover and start the full candida-cure diet.

WEEK ONE
Eliminate dairy products
(less dairy = less mucus and inflammation)

Check off items as you eliminate them:

	Check Off
Buttermilk	☐
Cheese (soft and hard)	☐
Cottage cheese	☐
Cow and goat milk (including nonfat, low fat, low lactose)	☐

	Check Off
Goat and sheep cheese (raw okay after 3 months)	☐
Ice cream	☐
Kefir	☐
Margarine	☐
Milk shakes	☐
Protein drinks, powders, or bars that contain dairy ingredients (cow's milk, whey)	☐
Sour cream	☐
Yogurt	☐

WEEK TWO
Eliminate refined carbohydrates and gluten
(fewer refined carbohydrates = less inflammation and plaque)

Check off items as you eliminate them:

	Check Off
Bagels	☐
Breads with yeast (sourdough, white, buns, rolls, etc.)	☐
Cereals (dry)	☐
Cookies	☐
Corn	☐
Crackers (wheat and white flour)	☐
Donuts	☐
Flour tortillas	☐
Gluten products (barley, kamut, oats, rye, spelt, triticale, wheat, white flour)	☐
Pasta (brown rice, buckwheat, and quinoa pasta are permitted once a week)	☐
Pastries	☐
Pizza	☐
White rice	☐

WEEK THREE
Eliminate sugar
(less sugar = less plaque,
pain, inflammation, and progression of MS)

Check off items as you eliminate them:

	Check Off
Agave nectar (Nectevia)	☐
Artificial sweeteners and sugar alcohols, such as aspartame (Nutrasweet), erythritol (Truvia, Nectresse), maltitol, mannitol, saccharin, sorbitol, and sucralose (Splenda)	☐
Barley malt	☐
Brown rice syrup	☐
Brown sugar	☐
Cakes, candy, cereals, chewing gum/lozenges (except with stevia, lo han, or xylitol), chocolate, cookies, donuts, ice cream, Jello and gelatins, pastries, pies, puddings	☐
Coconut sugar/nectar	☐
Corn syrup	☐
Dextrose	☐
Fruit-juice-sweetened products	☐
Fructose	☐
Honey (raw or processed)	☐
Maltodextrin	☐
Maple syrup	☐
Molasses	☐
Soft drinks, soda	☐
Sucanat, evaporated cane juice crystals, raw turbinado sugar	☐
Sucralose	☐
White sugar	☐
Yacon syrup	☐

WEEK FOUR
Eliminate miscellaneous foods

Check off items as you eliminate them:

	Check Off
Alcohol (including nonalcoholic beers because of their yeast content)	❏
Beans/legumes*	❏
Cashews*	❏
Coffee (caffeinated and decaffeinated)	❏
Condiments (ketchup, relish, pickles, soy sauce, jams, jellies, etc.)	❏
Energy drinks (e.g., Red Bull, vitamin waters)	❏
Hydrogenated oils in any food product (chips, margarine, breads, etc.)	❏
Kombucha	❏
Mushrooms	❏
Peanuts	❏
Pistachios*	❏
All fast foods (hamburgers with buns, fried foods, burritos, sandwiches, etc.)	❏
All fermented foods (miso, tempeh, soy sauce)	❏
All processed foods (TV dinners, bacon, beef jerky, bologna, pork sausage, etc.)	❏
All smoked, cured, dried, and pickled foods (bacon, bologna, smoked salmon)	❏
Soy (soy milk, tofu, soy protein powder, ponzu, miso, tamari, tempeh)	❏
Tobacco products and recreational drugs	❏

WEEK FIVE
Eliminate fruit
(less sugar = less plaque, pain, and inflammation)

Check off items as you eliminate them:

	Check Off
Apricots*	☐
Bananas*	☐
Cherries*	☐
Cranberries* (unsweetened after 3 months)	☐
Dried fruits (all—cranberries, dates, figs, raisins, prunes, etc.)	☐
Fruit juices (sweetened and unsweetened)	☐
Guavas*	☐
Grapes*	☐
Kiwis*	☐
Mangoes*	☐
Melons*	☐
Nectarines*	☐
Oranges*	☐
Papayas*	☐
Pineapples*	☐
Plums*	☐
Peaches*	☐
Pears*	☐
Persimmons*	☐
Pomegranates*	☐
Tangerines*	☐

CANDIDA-CURE DIET
MEAL IDEAS

The meal ideas below will show you just some of the possibilities for creating tasty meals while on the candida-cure diet. It's important to have a varied selection of foods so you don't get bored with the diet. Limit animal protein to no more than 4 ounces daily. You will find recipes for the starred (*) dishes in the Recipes section.

Be aware that some of these meals contain foods and ingredients that you may only eat after being on the diet for three months, so familiarize yourself with the "Foods to Eat" and "Foods to Avoid" lists.

Breakfast Ideas

- Eggs or egg whites prepared in a variety of ways with side of steamed spinach, cauliflower, or kale (soft-boiled, poached, hard-boiled, and sunny-side-up eggs are best; eat scrambled or omelets infrequently because of oxidized cholesterol from the yolks, or use egg whites only)

- Soft-boiled eggs with half a grapefruit

- Omelet with vegetables (avocado, spinach, and onion)

- Poached eggs with arugula or spinach: Layer pan with olive oil and large washed handful of spinach or arugula. Crack eggs on top of greens and poach (steam) until yolks are as desired.

- Hard-boiled egg with squirt of Basiltops dairy-free pesto (see www.basiltops.com)

- Egg scramble: Prepare with 2 egg whites, 2–3 spoonfuls of cooked quinoa or wild rice, a few squirts of Basiltops dairy-free pesto, and a handful of washed kale or spinach (sautéed until tender).

- Brown rice tortillas, Paleo Bread, or Sami's Millet & Flax Bread with nut butter, coconut butter, or tahini

- Egg sandwich/burrito: poached or sunny-side-up egg, Healthy Mayonnaise,* sliced red onion, and spinach leaves on a heated brown rice tortilla, Paleo Bread, Sami's Millet & Flax Bread, or lettuce leaf

- Hot cereal (amaranth, brown rice, buckwheat, or quinoa) with nuts, berries, a splash of almond or hemp milk, and sprinkle of cinnamon, sweetened with stevia, lo han, or xylitol if desired

- Turkey bacon or chicken sausage (antibiotic-, hormone- and gluten-free; if casing is pork, peel off after cooking) with sautéed vegetables

- Protein drink made with egg-white, hemp, or rice protein powder (no sugar). Blend with unsweetened almond, coconut, or hemp milk; one piece of fruit from "Foods to Eat" list; and 1 tsp of raw almond butter or coconut oil (melted) or raw nuts/seeds from "Foods to Eat" list.

- Ground turkey or chicken sautéed with diced sweet potatoes and onions

- Cold cereal: Lydia's Sprouted Cinnamon Cereal, Go Raw Simple Granola, or Qi'a Superfood – Chia, Buckwheat & Hemp Cereal (Nature's Path) with almond milk, pecans, berries, and cinnamon, sweetened with stevia, lo han, or xylitol if desired

- Vegetable Alkalizer Juice,* made with organic veggies

- Gluten-free waffles or pancakes, using Namaste Foods Waffle & Pancake Mix: Prepare with unsweetened almond, coconut, or hemp milk (sweeten with stevia, lo han, or xylitol if desired); top with mashed organic berries (blueberries, strawberries, raspberries, or blackberries); and garnish with sliced almonds and cinnamon.

- Amazing Meal Vanilla Chai Infusion (protein drink), mixed with 8 ounces of cold unsweetened almond milk

- Vegetable scramble (arugula, squash, onions, broccoli, and fresh herbs sautéed in olive oil) served over a bed of cooked millet or quinoa

- Leftover dinner from the night before

Lunch and Dinner Ideas

- Salad (greens: spinach, arugula, baby greens, and/or watercress; red onion; sprouts; sliced or grated carrots, jicama, radishes, and/or green apple; nuts, etc.) with Italian Vinaigrette Dressing*

- Black kale salad massaged with fresh lemon juice: Put in refrigerator for a couple of hours to soften kale and then add pine nuts, sea salt, and pepper.

- BLT salad (chopped romaine lettuce, diced avocado, cut-up cooked turkey bacon, diced jicama, and Ranch Dressing*)

- Cruciferous salad (cut-up spinach, watercress, parsley, avocado, red cabbage, green onions, cauliflower, and/or cucumber, topped with sesame seeds and Italian Vinaigrette Dressing*)

- Raw vegetable salad (shredded beets, zucchini, jicama, and chopped cucumber, topped with alfalfa sprouts and dressing)

- Chef's salad (baby greens, tomatoes, and cucumber, with diced cooked turkey, cut-up hard-boiled egg, and dressing)

- Greek salad (romaine lettuce, cut-up cooked chicken breast, olives, and lemon-dill dressing)

- Brown rice and steamed or sautéed vegetables, drizzled with olive oil, Real Salt, and other herbs or spices

- Buckwheat soba or kelp noodles in a stir-fry or with sautéed vegetables or chicken (use cold-pressed sesame oil and Bragg Liquid Aminos)

- Turkey burger with baked Sweet Potato Fries*

- Steamed vegetables topped with Macadamia Cream Sauce*

- Broiled, poached, or sautéed fish (salmon, cod, halibut, sole, trout, etc.) with side of sautéed greens

- Chicken salad on half an avocado

- Stews prepared in a Crock-Pot

- Baked vegetable medley: purple cabbage, kale, onion, red peppers, and brussels sprouts (toss vegetables in olive oil and herbs before baking), served over cooked millet

- Soups, non-dairy and sugar-free (vegetable, chicken vegetable, turkey, leek-broccoli puree, cauliflower-celery, carrot-celery-ginger, parsnip-butternut squash, etc.)

- Brown rice or quinoa pasta with fresh tomatoes, pine nuts, olive oil, garlic, and other vegetables if desired

- BLT wrap (cut-up cooked turkey bacon, lettuce, tomato, and avocado, with small amount of Healthy Mayonnaise*) in brown rice tortilla or lettuce leaf

- Turkey chili with side of mixed green salad (after 3 months)

- Stuffed zucchini or peppers (ground chicken or turkey, chopped onion, and seasonings) topped with marinara sauce

- Quinoa with vegetables and Basiltops dairy-free pesto

- Chicken or turkey tacos in brown rice tortillas or lettuce leaf, with guacamole, salsa, and shredded lettuce

- Chicken (broiled, roasted, baked, poached) with sautéed kale, cauliflower, and brussels sprouts

- Lamb or beef steak with sautéed onions, with side of sautéed asparagus

- Chicken or turkey sausage cut up and dipped in mustard, with side salad

- Vegetable stir-fry with or without chicken or fish (use cold-pressed sesame oil and Bragg Liquid Aminos)

- Roast chicken prepared with fresh herbs (thyme, rosemary), with side of roasted vegetables (purple cabbage, carrots, peppers, onions, kale—toss veggies in olive oil and seasoning before roasting)

- Turkey dogs (no nitrates, sugar, or dairy) with oven-baked turnip or parsnip fries (toss in grapeseed oil before baking)

- Turkey or chicken sandwich on gluten-, yeast-, dairy-, and sugar-free bread or lettuce wrap, with avocado, spinach, and mustard

- Egg salad sandwich on gluten-, yeast-, dairy-, and sugar-free bread or lettuce wrap (use Healthy Mayonnaise*)
- Lettuce wraps filled with diced chicken salad, wild rice, and slivered almonds
- Cornish Game Hen* stuffed with wild rice, with side cucumber salad (prepared with apple cider vinegar)
- Cabbage rolls stuffed with turkey, pumpkin, and brown rice
- Seaweed wraps filled with wild rice, chopped vegetable medley, and fresh-grated ginger (use organic nori sheets)

Side Dish Ideas

- Shredded slaw salad (raw purple and green cabbage and carrots with rice vinegar and seasonings)
- Collard greens or black kale sautéed in olive oil, with a splash of raw apple cider vinegar
- Sliced cucumbers with apple cider or rice vinegar and sea salt
- Wild rice pilaf made with organic chicken broth (no sugar)
- Mashed sweet potatoes made with almond milk and olive oil
- Artichokes with Dipping Sauce* (melted butter or Healthy Mayonnaise)
- Swiss chard, chopped and sautéed in olive oil, with pine nuts, fresh herbs, and sea salt
- Sautéed onions, peppers, and squashes
- Cold brown-rice salad with raw apple cider vinegar, vegetables, and seasonings
- Parsnips with butter (puree in blender)
- Asparagus sautéed in toasted sesame oil and sprinkled with sesame seeds
- Baked butternut squash with small amount of butter and stevia
- Quinoa with seasonings and spices or Basiltops dairy-free pesto

- Baked brussels sprouts and cauliflower with garlic, sea salt, and olive oil
- Millet with herbs and olive oil or tomato sauce
- Steamed broccoli and cauliflower with melted ghee or butter
- Amaranth with butter and seasonings
- Onions sautéed in olive oil
- Oven-baked turnip fries (toss in grapeseed oil before baking)
- Brown basmati rice sautéed in olive oil with cumin, topped with pine nuts or sliced almonds
- Fresh sprouts (broccoli, alfalfa, radish, sunflower) with fresh lemon juice or raw apple cider vinegar
- Radish and fennel salad with fresh dill and rice vinegar
- Oven-roasted vegetables (squash, onions, carrots, red cabbage) seasoned with thyme and rosemary (toss in olive oil before roasting)

Snacks and Desserts

- Sami's Millet & Flax Bread or Paleo Bread with almond or coconut butter or sesame seed tahini, a drop of stevia, and sprinkle of cinnamon
- Hard-boiled egg with mustard
- Kale Chips*
- Brown-rice cakes or flax crackers with nut/seed butter (almond, macadamia nut, sunflower seed, or pumpkin seed) or coconut butter
- Cut-up vegetables (carrot sticks, broccoli, jicama, celery) dipped in Tahini Sauce,* Ranch Dressing,* or Guacamole*
- Garlic spread (Majestic Garlic) on flax crisps or crusts (Mauk Family Farms' Raw Wheat Free or Raw Mineral Rich Crusts)
- Celery with almond butter, macadamia nut butter, sunflower seed butter, or pumpkin seed butter

- Fruit from the "Foods to Eat" list, one piece (or a handful of berries)
- Pumpkin or acorn squash slices (baked with olive oil, cinnamon, and sea salt)
- Baked apple with cinnamon and nuts
- Carob or raw cacao muffins (Namaste sugar-free Muffin Mix: add eggs, nuts, berries, unsweetened raw cacao or carob powder, stevia or xylitol (carob and cacao okay only after 3 months)
- Cookies and treats made without gluten, dairy, or sugar (such as Nutty Nibbles by Nut Just a Cookie, sugar-free variety). Or make your own using gluten-free flours; coconut flour; almond meal; butter, ghee, or coconut oil; nut butters; and sweeteners such as stevia, lo han, chicory root, or xylitol.
- Smoothie made with egg-white protein powder (Vitol, vanilla), almond milk, blueberries, and nut butter (or melted coconut oil or coconut butter); see Blueberry Buckle shake in Recipes section
- Cacao bars (Rox Chox, made with xylitol; after 3 months)
- DNA Life Bars (after 3 months; made with sweet potato, pumpkin, oats, and xylitol)

Sauces and Seasonings

- Salsa* (without sugar or vinegar, except raw apple cider vinegar)
- Guacamole* (avocados, tomatoes, onion, and spices)
- Sesame-ginger-garlic sauce, made with cold-pressed sesame oil, ginger, and garlic
- Lemon-garlic sauce, made with olive oil, garlic, and lemon juice (use over gluten-free pasta)
- Fresh-squeezed lemon or lime juice
- Bragg Liquid Aminos (unfermented soy sauce; salty flavor is good for stir-fries)

- Italian Vinaigrette Dressing*
- Unsweetened orange or pineapple juice as a marinade for fish or chicken (these fruits are acceptable only for marinade)
- Healthy Mayonnaise*
- Bragg Organic Sea Kelp Delight Seasoning
- Seaweed flakes
- Curry (coconut milk, turmeric, cumin, ginger, and garlic paste)
- Raw Coconut Aminos (use like soy sauce; www.coconutsecret.com)
- Macadamia Cream Sauce*
- Spices—cayenne, turmeric, ginger, cumin, epazote, coriander, curry, cinnamon, bay leaves, basil, etc.

TWO WEEKS OF
SAMPLE MENUS

The two weeks' worth of sample menus that follow will give you an idea of the diverse menus you can create while on the candida-cure diet. You will find recipes for the starred (*) dishes in the Recipes section, which also includes recipes not listed here.

WEEK ONE

Day One

Upon arising	1 cup of red clover tea
Breakfast	Poached egg with side of sautéed vegetables (onions and kale), topped with slices of avocado
Snack	Apple (green) with a small handful of raw almonds
Lunch	Amaranth Tabouli*
Snack	Vegetable Alkalizer Juice* (8 ounces)
Dinner	Salmon with dill-lemon juice
	Baby greens salad with Italian Vinaigrette Dressing*

Day Two

Upon arising	1 cup of red clover tea
Breakfast	Vegetable hash (diced onions, spinach, parsnips, and fresh herbs sautéed in olive oil)
Snack	Blueberries topped with coconut butter
Lunch	Brown rice and vegetable stir-fry (see Chicken Stir-Fry recipe)
Snack	Jicama slices dipped in Zesty Tahini Sauce*

Dinner	Tuscan Roast Chicken*
	Artichoke* with melted butter
	Sautéed squash in olive oil and herbs

Day Three

Upon arising	1 cup of red clover tea
Breakfast	Cold cereal (Qi'a Superfood – Chia, Buckwheat & Hemp, original flavor) with berries, unsweetened almond, coconut, or hemp milk and lo han, stevia, or xylitol to sweeten
Snack	Cut-up raw vegetables (broccoli, carrots, jicama, asparagus) with Ranch Dressing*
Lunch	African-Style Turkey*
	Spinach, red onion, and sprout salad with Italian Vinaigrette Dressing*
Snack	Handful of Spicy Almonds*
	1 cup of red clover tea
Dinner	Kelp noodles or quinoa pasta with garlic, pine nuts, basil, and vegetables

Day Four

Upon arising	1 cup of red clover tea
Breakfast	Cinnamon Buckwheat Hot Cereal* with 1 tbsp ground flaxseed, raspberries, cinnamon, and a splash of almond milk
Snack	Vegetable Alkalizer Juice* (8 ounces)
Lunch	Chicken fajitas with sautéed vegetables, guacamole, and salsa on a lettuce wrap or brown rice tortilla
Snack	Olive Tapenade* on flax crackers
	1 cup of red clover tea
Dinner	Vegetable soup with quinoa

Day Five

Upon arising	1 cup of red clover tea
Breakfast	Egg sandwich (sunny-side-up egg on lettuce wrap with Healthy Mayonnaise,* sprouts, avocado, and sesame seeds)
Snack	Celery sticks with sunflower seed butter
	1 cup of red clover tea
Lunch	Sweetened Butternut Squash*
	Arugula, Beet, and Walnut Salad*
Snack	Vegetable Alkalizer Juice* (8 ounces)
Dinner	Cod with Macadamia Nut Sauce*
	Sautéed brussels sprouts and black kale and/or collard greens

Day Six

Upon arising	2 cups of red clover tea
Breakfast	Blueberry-Strawberry Pancakes*
Snack	Green apple with almond butter
Lunch	Quinoa Medley*
	Cucumber Salad*
Snack	Kale chips
	1 cup of red clover tea
Dinner	Ground turkey burger (with mustard, baby greens, avocado, and sautéed onion) wrapped in lettuce leaf
	Side of sliced raw broccoli and cucumbers with Zesty Tahini Sauce*

Day Seven

Upon arising	2 cups of red clover tea
Breakfast	Vegetable scramble with diced squash,

	cauliflower, mustard greens, chives, and cooked quinoa
Snack	Guacamole with cut-up vegetables
Lunch	Seared halibut salad with Wasabi-Ginger Dressing*
Snack	Tahini Toast*
Dinner	Cornish Game Hen* stuffed with wild rice Side of steamed spinach
Dessert	Baked Apple* with cinnamon

WEEK TWO

Day One

Upon arising	2 cups of red clover tea
Breakfast	Protein Smoothie*
Snack	Half a grapefruit
Lunch	Trout with Ginger-Wasabi Dressing* Grilled asparagus with toasted sesame seeds Citrus Soda*
Snack	Half an avocado with a sprinkle of sea salt 1 cup of red clover tea
Dinner	Quinoa Burger* Asian Coleslaw*

Day Two

Upon arising	2 cups of red clover tea
Breakfast	Rice-Almond Pancakes*
Snack	Vegetable Alkalizer Juice* (8 ounces)
Lunch	Chicken Soup*
Snack	Celery and carrot sticks with Ranch Dressing* 2 cups of red clover tea
Dinner	Fish Curry* over brown basmati rice Marinated Kale Salad*

Day Three

Upon arising	2 cups of red clover tea
Breakfast	Arugula and tomato salad topped with grilled onions, turkey bacon, and poached egg, drizzled with olive oil, sea salt, and pepper
Snack	Cucumber slices and sprouts with raw apple cider vinegar
Lunch	Indian Risotto*
Snack	Pumpkin seeds (small handful)
	2 cups of red clover tea
Dinner	Turkey Meatloaf*
	Mashed Faux-tatoes*
	Side salad

Day Four

Upon arising	2 cups of red clover tea
Breakfast	Qi'a Superfood cereal with almond, coconut, or hemp milk, topped with berries and sliced almonds, and sweetened with xylitol or stevia
Snack	Flax crackers with pumpkin seed butter
Lunch	Spaghetti Squash with Parsley Pesto Sauce*
Snack	Green apple with small handful of walnuts
	2 cups of red clover tea
Dinner	Roast Duckling*
	Leeks and Leaves*

Day Five

Upon arising	2 cups of red clover tea
Breakfast	Hard-boiled egg with squirt of Basiltops dairy-free pesto
Snack	Handful of Spicy Almonds*
Lunch	Mixed baby-greens salad topped with baked vegetables (peppers, asparagus, zucchini,

and yellow squash tossed in olive oil with
fresh thyme, sea salt, and pepper)

Snack   Handful of blackberries
               2 cups of red clover tea
Dinner   Cod with Olive Tapenade*
               Shredded beet and watercress salad sprinkled
               with toasted pine nuts and Italian Vinaigrette*

Day Six

Upon arising   2 cups of red clover tea
Breakfast   Amazing Meal Vanilla Chai Infusion mixed
               with 8 oz. of cold unsweetened almond milk
Snack   Jicama with Ranch Dressing*
Lunch   BLT salad (chopped romaine lettuce, diced
               avocado, cut-up cooked turkey bacon,
               diced jicama, and Ranch Dressing*)
Snack   Blueberry Buckle Shake*
               2 cups of red clover tea
Dinner   Buckwheat soba noodles with vegetables

Day Seven

Upon arising   2 cups of red clover tea
Breakfast   Ground chicken with vegetables
               (diced cauliflower, peppers, garlic, kale)
Snack   Vegetable Alkalizer Juice* (8 ounces)
Lunch   Wild rice pilaf with sautéed asparagus,
               purple cabbage, and onions
Snack   Sweet Potato or Parsnip Fries*
               2 cups of red clover tea
Dinner   Watercress, fennel, avocado, and sliced green
               apple salad with Cumin Vinaigrette*
Dessert   Pumpkin Pie*

RECIPES

This section will help get you started creating meals that fit within the parameters of your candida-cure diet. You can also experiment with your own ideas, using these recipes as a guideline.

Whenever possible, use free-range, antibiotic-free, and hormone-free beef, chicken, turkey, and eggs. Buy wild-caught fish instead of farmed, and use organic vegetables and fruits whenever possible. Stay away from genetically modified foods. Unless packaged foods specifically state that the product or ingredients are non-GMO or organic, you can assume that they're not. Make sure your mustard is made with apple cider vinegar rather than other types of vinegar, and use purified water for cooking. Whenever a recipe calls for olive oil, use cold-pressed organic extra-virgin olive oil.

Please be aware that some of the recipe ingredients should not be used until you have strictly adhered to the "Foods to Avoid" list for at least three months. Xylitol powder (Ultimate Sweetener by Ultimate Life), chicory root (Just Like Sugar), or lo han (Lo Han Sweet by Jarrow) may be substituted for stevia wherever that is called for.

MAIN DISHES

Turkey Quinoa Meatloaf

- 1 lb ground organic turkey
- 2 eggs
- ¼ cup uncooked quinoa
- 1 medium onion, finely chopped
- 3 garlic cloves, finely chopped
- 2 chilies, finely chopped
- 1 tbsp coconut oil or olive oil
- 1 tsp thyme

    1 tsp rosemary
    ¼ tsp black pepper
    1 tsp sea salt

Cook quinoa as directed on page 288. Preheat oven to 350°F. Chop onion, chilies, and garlic cloves finely or in a food processor. Add cooked quinoa and all ingredients to a large bowl and mix together. Grease a loaf pan with coconut or olive oil, add the mixture, and bake for 1 hour.

Spaghetti Squash with Parsley Pesto Sauce

    1 medium organic spaghetti squash
    2 cups loosely packed fresh organic Italian parsley, large stems removed (don't discard)
    ½ cup roasted macadamia or pine nuts
    2 garlic cloves, minced
    2 tsp lemon juice
    1 tsp lime juice
    ½ cup olive oil
    ½ tsp sea salt
       cilantro, chopped (for garnish)

1. Preheat oven to 375°.
2. Pierce spaghetti squash shell several times with a fork, and place in an oiled baking dish. Bake 25 minutes, turn squash over, and bake until flesh is tender and yields gently to pressure, approximately 20–30 minutes more.
3. While squash is cooking, strip parsley leaves from the stems and set leaves aside. Finely chop the stems and place in a blender or food processor.
4. To make pesto sauce, add nuts, garlic, lemon and lime juices, oil, and sea salt to blender/food processor and puree. Add the parsley leaves and process until they are coarsely chopped.
5. Once squash is cooked, let cool 10–15 minutes, then cut in half and use a spoon to remove seeds and strings from the center. Gently scrape the tines of a kitchen fork around the

edge of the spaghetti squash to shred the pulp into "spaghetti" strands.

6. Put spaghetti into a large bowl, add pesto sauce, and mix well. Sprinkle with chopped cilantro leaves and serve.

Spicy Chicken and Cabbage Soup

- 2 tbsp olive oil
- 1 large onion, diced
- 2 medium carrots, diced
- 2 celery stalks, diced
- 4 cloves garlic, minced
- 8 cups chicken stock (preferably homemade)
- 4 chicken breasts, skin removed
- 1¾ lbs sauce tomatoes, whole (Roma or dry-farmed Early Girl)
- 1 tsp paprika
- 1 tsp garlic granules
- ½ tsp dried thyme
- ½ tsp dried oregano
- ½ tsp black pepper
- ½ tsp cayenne pepper
- 1 large head green cabbage, cored and coarsely chopped
  Sea salt to taste

Heat the oil in a large stockpot over medium heat. Add onion, carrots, celery, garlic, and a pinch of sea salt. Cook, stirring frequently, until onion is translucent, about 8 minutes. Add chicken stock, chicken breasts, tomatoes, paprika, garlic granules, thyme, oregano, black pepper, and cayenne pepper. Bring to a boil, then reduce heat and simmer, covered, for 20 minutes. Remove the chicken from the pot and strip the meat from the bones. Cut the meat into bite-size pieces. Return the chicken to the pot, add the cabbage, and mix well, breaking up the tomatoes. Add water if the soup is too crowded. Bring to a boil once again. Reduce the heat and simmer, covered, for another 15 minutes. Season with sea salt to taste.

Pico de Gallo Omelet

4 eggs
   Splash of hemp, almond, or coconut milk
1 avocado, sliced
1 cup Pico de Gallo Sauce

Pico De Gallo Sauce

¼ cup onion, chopped
1 large tomato
¼ cup cilantro, chopped
   Squeeze of fresh lime juice
¼ cup jalapeños, chopped

Beat eggs and milk together. Cook as an omelet. Fill with avocado and Pico de Gallo Sauce.

Cabbage Rolls

1 lb ground white turkey meat
1 tbsp olive oil
¼ cup onion, chopped
¼ cup toasted pine nuts
   Dash of cayenne
   Sea salt and pepper to taste
½ cup fresh tomato, pureed
4–6 green cabbage leaves
8 oz vegetable broth

Rinse and dry cabbage leaves and steam for 3 minutes. While they are cooling, sauté turkey meat, onion, and spices in olive oil until turkey is lightly browned. Add tomato puree and cook over medium heat for about 10 minutes, stirring occasionally. Let cool. Mix in toasted pine nuts. Pour vegetable broth into a baking dish. Fill each leaf with turkey mixture, fold over, and place in the baking dish. Cover with foil and bake at 325° for 30 minutes.

Egg Salad

2 hard-boiled eggs
1 tbsp mayonnaise
¼ cup onion, chopped
  Sea salt and pepper to taste

Mix all ingredients.

Chicken Salad

2 boneless chicken breasts, cubed and baked (without skin)
¼ cup pecans (raw), chopped
½ tsp dill, freshly minced
1½ tbsp mayonnaise
  Sea salt and pepper to taste

Mix all ingredients.

Homemade Chicken Soup

2 large chicken breasts, including bones and skin
1 clove garlic, peeled
1 tbsp olive oil
1 4-oz can of tomato sauce
½ cup carrots, sliced
2 stalks celery, diced (add tops as well for flavor)
1 bunch kale, chopped
1 large yellow onion, chopped
2–3 quarts water
  Sea salt and pepper to taste

Place all ingredients in a 6-quart stock pot. Bring to a boil, and then simmer on low for 3 hours, stirring occasionally.

Fish Curry

1 tsp Thai Kitchen red or green curry paste
1 cup coconut milk, unsweetened
1 tsp fresh lime juice

  3   stalks of lemongrass, cut into quarters
1–1½ lbs fresh white fish of your choice, cut into chunks

Combine coconut milk, lime juice, lemongrass, and curry paste in a skillet. Simmer on low for 5 minutes. Add fish. Cook on low for 5–10 minutes. Do not eat pieces of lemongrass, as they are too sharp and chewy.

Chicken Stir-Fry

  1   tbsp coconut oil
  ½   cup broccoli florets, cut into bite-size pieces
  ½   cup carrots, sliced
  ¼   cup water chestnuts
  4   oz boneless and skinless chicken tenders, cubed
  ½   cup onion, sliced
  ¾   cup bok choy, chopped
  1   tbsp Bragg Liquid Aminos
      Toasted sesame seeds

Place wok or skillet over medium heat. Add coconut oil and heat for 3 minutes. Add the rest of the ingredients, except the sesame seeds. Stir-fry on high heat for 5–10 minutes. Cook until vegetables are the desired texture. Top with sesame seeds and serve.

Cornish Game Hens

  1   cup wild rice, cooked
  1   tsp olive oil
  ¼   tsp fresh thyme, finely chopped
  ¼   tsp fresh sage, finely chopped
  ¼   tsp fresh rosemary, finely chopped
  ½   cup toasted pine nuts
  2   Cornish game hens
  1   onion, peeled and thinly sliced
  5   garlic cloves, peeled and halved
      Sea salt and pepper to taste
      Butter (melted) and olive oil for basting

Cook wild rice as directed on package to make 1 cup of cooked rice. Mix in olive oil, herbs, and toasted pine nuts. Stuff game hens with rice mixture and place in a roasting pan. Scatter onions and garlic around the outside of the hens. Brush hens with melted butter and olive oil, and season with salt and pepper. Bake at 375° for 1 hour, basting occasionally.

Brown Rice Penne with Chicken Sausage and Vegetables

- 8 oz brown rice penne
- 2 chicken sausage links (peel off pork casings after cooking)
- ½ red bell pepper, diced
- 3 Roma tomatoes, diced
- 1 cup fresh arugula, washed and finely chopped
- 1 tbsp olive oil

Cook brown rice penne in boiling salted water as directed on package. Broil chicken sausage links until cooked. Peel off pork casings when cooled. Slice links and put aside. In a large saucepan, heat olive oil and add bell peppers and tomatoes. Sauté for 10 minutes. Add arugula and cook until wilted. Remove from heat, mix in sliced sausage and penne, and serve.

Quinoa Burger*

- 1 medium onion, chopped
- 3 garlic cloves, minced
- 1 tbsp olive oil
- 1 cup cooked black beans
- 1 carrot, finely grated
- ½ cup baked sweet potato (without skin)
- 1 cup cooked quinoa (see recipe below)
- 1 tbsp caraway seeds
- 3 tbsp cilantro, chopped
- 2 tbsp tomato paste
- 1 tsp raw apple cider vinegar

*Avoid for first three months.

Pinch of cayenne (optional)
Pinch of sea salt

Sauté onions and garlic in 1 tbsp of olive oil. Add beans and cook for 2 minutes. Turn off heat and mash beans in pan. Put beans into a bowl and mix in remaining ingredients. Form patties and bake until heated through, approximately 5–10 minutes on each side.

QUINOA

Soak ¼ cup of raw quinoa for 15 minutes, if possible, to remove the saponin coating, which can have a bitter taste. Rinse quinoa thoroughly. In a saucepan, bring to a boil ½ cup of water, ¼ cup of quinoa, and a pinch of sea salt. Cover and simmer for about 20 minutes. Remove from heat and allow to sit for 5 minutes.

Indian Risotto*

   1 tbsp ghee (clarified butter)
   1 jalapeño, minced
   1 tsp cumin seeds
   ⅛ tsp asafetida
   1 cup split yellow mung beans, uncooked
   1 cup brown basmati rice, rinsed well in 3 changes of water
   1 small cauliflower, cut into florets
   6 cups water
   ½ tsp ground turmeric
  1½ tsp sea salt
      Fresh ground pepper to taste

Heat ½ tbsp of ghee in a saucepan. Add jalapeño and cumin seeds. Cook until seeds begin to darken. Add asafetida and stir for a minute. Then add mung beans, rice, and cauliflower, and cook for 3 minutes while stirring. Add 4½ cups of water, turmeric, and salt, and bring to a boil. Lower heat, cover, and simmer, stirring frequently, until the beans and rice are tender (30–40 minutes). Add more water if necessary. Stir in black pepper and drizzle with remaining melted ghee.

*Avoid for first three months.

Tuscan Country Roast Chicken

1 roasting chicken, 3 lbs or more, thawed
    Bay leaves to taste (4 fresh or 2 dry)
½ lemon (with peel)
    Several garlic cloves, halved
    Sea salt and fresh ground pepper

Preheat oven to 400°. Rinse chicken and wipe dry. Fill cavity with bay leaves, lemon, salt, pepper, and a couple of garlic cloves. Salt and pepper chicken on all sides. Tuck remaining garlic clove halves into the hollows of the thighs and wings. Place chicken on a rack in a roasting pan with about 1 inch of water in the bottom to keep drippings from burning. Bake at 400° for 90 minutes. Reduce temperature to 350° and bake for 15–30 minutes or until legs move easily and juices run clear.

Optional: Make gravy with pan juices, and pour over a whole grain of your choice.

Roast Duckling

1 4–5 lb duckling, completely defrosted
    Chef's Salt (see recipe below)
4 tbsp butter
1 parsnip or carrot, chopped
2 stalks celery, chopped
1 onion, chopped
2 garlic cloves, thinly sliced
4 black peppercorns
1 bay leaf
½ tsp marjoram

CHEF'S SALT

½ cup sea salt
½ tbsp paprika
½ tsp black pepper
1 tsp white pepper

1   tsp celery salt
1   tsp garlic salt (not powder)

Mix all ingredients for Chef's Salt. Preheat oven to 300°. Spread butter in the bottom of a roasting pan that has a tight-fitting lid. Remove neck and giblets from duck cavity and discard. Rinse duck in cold water and rub inside and out with Chef's Salt. Place duck, breast-side down, directly on the butter in the roasting pan. Place vegetables and garlic inside and around the duckling. Add about 2 inches of water to the pan. Add the peppercorns and bay leaf, and sprinkle marjoram on the duck and in the water. Cover and cook for 2 hours. Carefully remove duckling to a platter and let it cool (if you don't let it cool, it won't turn out right). Split duckling lengthwise by standing it on the neck end and cutting with a sharp knife from the tip of the tail down the center. Quarter if desired. Save leftovers for soup.

Turkey Soup with Winter Vegetables

1 or 2   large turkey legs
2   bay leaves
1   tsp dried parsley
1   tsp dried thyme
1   daikon radish *or*
2   carrots, chopped
1   large parsnip, chopped
2   turnips, chopped
3   stalks celery, chopped
1   yellow onion, chopped
    Sea salt and pepper to taste

Place turkey legs in a large soup pot. Cover with purified water. Add bay leaves, parsley, and thyme and bring to a boil. Simmer for 4 hours, until meat falls off the bones. Strain soup and remove bones. Dice meat and add back into the broth. Add vegetables and simmer for 1 more hour. Salt and pepper to taste.

African-Style Turkey

2 lbs boneless, skinless turkey breasts, cut into bite-size pieces
½ cup chicken or vegetable broth
1 large onion, chopped
4 garlic cloves, minced
½ tsp crushed red pepper flakes
1 tsp fresh ginger, minced or grated
1 tsp sea salt
¼ tsp black pepper
1 tbsp fresh lemon juice

Place all ingredients in a large, covered pot and cook for 45 minutes to 1 hour on low heat. Serve over a whole grain of your choosing.

Marinated Tri-Tip Roast

1 1½–2 lb tri-tip roast
½ tbsp sea salt
½ tbsp cracked black peppercorns
1 tbsp minced garlic cloves
1 tbsp fresh ginger root, grated
1 tbsp Bragg Liquid Aminos
½ tbsp white pepper
5 drops of stevia

Mix all ingredients well and cover the meat with them. Place the meat and any excess marinade in a plastic storage bag and put in the refrigerator for at least an hour or, better, overnight. Place meat in a roasting pan and cover it with remaining marinade from the plastic bag. Roast at 425° for 30–35 minutes. When the meat is cooked to desired doneness, carve across the grain into thin slices.

SIDE DISHES

Mashed Faux-tatoes

1 large head of cauliflower
¾ cup unsalted chicken stock (preferably homemade)
2 tbsp unsalted butter
   Sea salt to taste

Wash cauliflower and cut into pieces. Combine cauliflower and chicken stock in a 2-quart pan. Bring to a boil and then reduce heat. Simmer, covered, until cauliflower is tender, about 20 minutes. Remove from heat, but do not drain the liquid! Mix the butter in and let it melt. Puree the mixture in the pan using an immersion blender. Add sea salt to taste and mix well again.

Artichokes with Dipping Sauce

1 artichoke per serving
1 bay leaf
   Pinch of sea salt
1 tbsp Healthy Mayonnaise per serving (see p. 297)

Wash artichokes. Cut off stems to base and stand upright in a large saucepan. Add 2–3 inches of water to the pan. Add the bay leaf and sprinkle the sea salt into the water. Cover and simmer over medium heat until the base is tender—about 45 minutes. Add more water if needed. Use Healthy Mayonnaise as dipping sauce.

Stir-Fried Asparagus

10–12 spears of asparagus
4 tbsp olive oil
3 tbsp sesame oil
6 garlic cloves, minced
½ tsp sea salt
   Crushed red pepper to taste

Heat wok or skillet over medium heat. After 1 minute, add oils and heat for 1 minute. Add asparagus and turn heat to high. Stir-fry for 5 minutes or until asparagus are seared, or lightly browned. Add garlic, salt, and red pepper, and stir-fry for about 2 more minutes. Serve hot.

Broccoli with Sliced Almonds

1 large head broccoli cut into small florets
¼ cup raw sliced almonds
2 tbsp olive oil
Sea salt and pepper to taste

Steam broccoli for 7 minutes. Dry-fry almonds in skillet over low heat for 2–3 minutes; then add olive oil and broccoli. Sauté for 2–3 minutes, adding sea salt and pepper to taste.

Sweetened Butternut Squash

1 butternut squash
1 tbsp butter
⅓ cup chopped pecans or walnuts
Spices to your liking (cinnamon, nutmeg, or pumpkin pie spice)
Pinch of powdered stevia

Cut squash in half. Place cut-side down in a pan with ¼ inch of water. Bake at 375° for 1 hour or until soft. Scoop out desired amount of squash flesh and top with butter, nuts, and spices to taste.

Arugula, Beet, and Walnut Salad

1 large bunch arugula, washed well (discard stems)
¼ cup red onion, chopped
½ cup tomatoes, diced
1 apple, diced
¼ cup beets, cooked and diced
¼ cup walnuts, raw or dry-roasted in 350° oven for 10 mins.
Italian Vinaigrette Dressing (see page 296)

Southern Greens Mix

2 cups mixed collard greens, chard, and mustard greens
1 tbsp olive oil
1 tbsp raw apple cider vinegar
1 tsp raw, hulled sesame seeds
  Pinch of sea salt

Heat skillet. Add olive oil and heat for one minute. Add kale and sauté over low heat until tender. Add the remaining vegetables and ingredients, and sauté for another 3 minutes.

Marinated Kale Salad

3–4 cups black kale, shredded
2 tomatoes, diced
1 carrot, grated
¼ cup red onion, diced
½ avocado, diced
  Vinaigrette Dressing

VINAIGRETTE DRESSING

¾ cup raw apple cider vinegar
¼ cup toasted sesame oil or olive oil
3 garlic cloves, minced
1 tsp mustard powder

Toss the kale and vegetables (not the avocado) with the vinaigrette dressing. Marinate for at least 4 hours or overnight in refrigerator so vegetables become tender. Add avocado when ready to eat.

Asian Coleslaw

2–3 cups cabbage, chopped
¼ cup daikon radish, grated
¾ cup green onions, finely chopped
1 green apple, finely chopped
1 cup sliced raw almonds or sunflower seeds
2 tbsp raw, hulled sesame seeds

Sea salt and pepper to taste
Coleslaw dressing

Coleslaw Dressing

¼ cup sesame oil
¼ cup rice vinegar (unseasoned, unsweetened)
2 tbsp fresh lemon juice
1–3 drops of stevia liquid

Put all ingredients in a jar and shake well. Pour over coleslaw mixture. Season with salt and pepper.

Candied Yam

1 small yam
Butter
1–3 drops of stevia liquid

Bake yam at 350° until tender, about 45 minutes. Slice open and add butter and stevia.

Sweet Potato or Parsnip Fries

2 sweet potatoes or 3 large parsnips, sliced like French fries
2 tbsp grapeseed oil
Sea salt

Put sliced sweet potatoes (or parsnips) in a bowl. Pour grapeseed oil over them and mix to make sure oil covers all sides. Lay out fries on a baking sheet and sprinkle with sea salt. Bake at 400° for 45 minutes. After 20 minutes, turn fries over to cook on the other side.

Leeks and Leaves

6 leeks
2–3 tbsp butter
½–1 cup vegetable stock (use larger amount if you like a soupier mixture)
1–2 bunches spinach, chard, or kale, or a mixture, chopped

Pinch of nutmeg
Sea salt to taste

Trim the leeks, using only the white and pale green parts. Slice in half lengthwise, wash well, and dry. Slice crosswise into small pieces. Sauté leeks in butter in a large skillet until they soften and begin to fall apart. Add stock and season lightly with sea salt and nutmeg. Stir and simmer for 5 minutes. Add greens and simmer until cooked.

SAUCES, DRESSINGS, AND DIPS

Italian Vinaigrette Dressing

¾ cup olive oil
¼–½ cup raw, unfiltered apple cider vinegar
2 stalks rosemary sprigs
1 cup fresh basil, chopped
3 garlic cloves, peeled and mashed
1 tsp dry mustard (optional)
1–2 drops stevia liquid or ¼ tsp stevia powder (optional)

Put all ingredients in a jar and shake well. Keep refrigerated.

Cumin Vinaigrette

½ cup olive oil
1 tsp Eden Foods Organic Yellow (or Brown) Mustard
½ tsp ground cumin
½ tsp minced garlic
2½ tbsp raw apple cider vinegar

Put all ingredients in a jar and shake well. Keep refrigerated.

Ranch Dressing

1 cup whole, raw macadamia nuts (soak for 1–2 hours; rinse and drain)
½ fresh lemon, squeezed
1 tsp sea salt

 1 tbsp fresh chives
 1 tsp fresh or dried parsley
 1 garlic clove *or* 1 tsp garlic powder
 1 tsp fresh dill
 ¼ tsp black pepper
 ⅓ cup olive oil
    Pinch of cayenne (optional)
    Purified water, as needed

Blend all ingredients in blender until smooth. Add enough water to achieve the desired consistency.

Ginger-Wasabi Dressing

 1 tbsp ginger, freshly grated
 ¼ tsp fresh horseradish root, grated
 ¼ cup rice vinegar, unsweetened
 1 tsp sea salt

Healthy Mayonnaise

 1 egg
 1 tsp Eden Foods Organic Yellow (or Brown) Mustard
 1 tbsp raw, unfiltered apple cider vinegar *or* fresh lemon juice
 ¼ tsp sea salt
 ¾ cup grapeseed oil or sunflower seed oil

Put egg, mustard, vinegar or lemon juice, and sea salt in blender or food processor. Blend until smooth. Slowly add in oil and pulse until smooth and creamy.

Zesty Tahini Sauce

 ¼ cup raw tahini
 2 drops stevia liquid *or* ¼ tsp stevia powder (optional)
    Purified water and/or fresh lemon juice if needed to achieve desired consistency
    Pinch of cayenne

No-Cheese Pesto

3 cups fresh basil
¾ cup olive oil
1 tsp sea salt
4 garlic cloves, peeled
½ cup dry-roasted pine nuts
2 tbsp fresh lemon juice

Blend all ingredients in blender and serve over vegetables or brown rice pasta.

Olive Tapenade

½ cup black olives, pitted and chopped
3 tbsp fresh lemon juice
1 tbsp olive oil
1 tsp sea salt
¼ cup dry-roasted pine nuts, finely chopped

Hand mix all ingredients.

Guacamole

1 medium-sized ripe avocado, peeled and pitted
4 tsp fresh lemon juice
1 tsp onion, finely chopped
Sea salt to taste
Fresh cilantro, chopped (optional)

Mash avocado and mix in remaining ingredients.

Salsa

2 cups tomatoes, diced
1 tbsp olive oil
1 medium onion, chopped
1 tbsp fresh lemon juice
1 jalapeño, finely chopped
Sea salt and pepper to taste

Hand mix all ingredients.

Macadamia Cream Sauce

15 raw macadamia nuts
½ tsp sea salt
    Juice of ½ fresh lemon
¼ cup basil, chopped
1 garlic clove

Blend all ingredients in blender. Add more lemon juice if needed to achieve desired consistency. Use on vegetables and grains.

Tahini Dressing

3 tbsp tahini
1 tbsp raw, unfiltered apple cider vinegar
4 tbsp olive oil or flaxseed oil
3 tbsp fresh lemon juice
2–3 drops stevia
    Seasonings as desired (fresh garlic or garlic powder, sea salt, pepper, pinch of cayenne)

Put all ingredients in a jar and shake well. Keep refrigerated.

GRAINS

Rice-Almond Pancakes

1½ cups brown rice flour
¼ cup almond flour
1 egg
¼ cup almond milk
¼ tsp cinnamon
⅔ cup water
4 drops or ½ tsp stevia
    Dash of vanilla extract (alcohol-free)

Combine all ingredients to desired consistency (more liquid equals thinner pancakes). Butter skillet and cook until golden brown.

Blueberry Muffins

1½ cups Namaste Muffin Mix (sugar-free)
½–1 cup organic blueberries or raspberries
1 tsp baking soda
½ tsp nutmeg
2 tsp cinnamon
1 tsp vanilla extract (alcohol-free)
2 eggs
2 tbsp water
½ cup butter, softened
1½ cup chopped pecans

Heat oven to 350°. Lightly oil muffin tin or insert paper liners. Combine all ingredients in large bowl. Fill tins to top with batter. Bake 14–16 minutes or until toothpick inserted in center comes out clean.

Blueberry-Strawberry Pancakes

2 cups Namaste Foods Waffle & Pancake Mix
2 eggs
2 tablespoons coconut oil, melted
⅛ cup raw sliced almonds
½ cup water or unsweetened almond, coconut, or hemp milk
¼ cup blueberries
   Pinch of cinnamon or nutmeg
¼ cup strawberries (wash and cut tops off, mash into a puree with fork, and sweeten with small amount of xylitol or stevia)
   Butter or grapeseed oil

Combine eggs, melted coconut oil, nuts, water or milk substitute, blueberries, cinnamon/nutmeg, and Namaste mix, and mix well. Add more liquid if you desire thinner pancakes. Preheat pan with butter or grapeseed oil on low to medium heat. Add batter and cook to desired doneness. Top with pureed strawberries.

Sesame Millet

    1   cup uncooked millet
    3   cups water
    1   tsp sea salt
    2   tbsp olive oil
    ¼   cup raw, hulled sesame seeds

Wash millet and drain. Boil water and add sea salt. Add millet, cover, and simmer on low heat for 25–30 minutes. Let stand for 5–10 minutes to increase fluffiness. While millet is standing, put sesame seeds into a frying pan and toast over low flame for 5 minutes, stirring frequently until golden brown. Once seeds are brown, add olive oil and millet. Stir mixture over medium heat for 5 minutes and serve.

Quinoa Medley

    2   cups uncooked quinoa
    ⅔   cup red bell peppers, finely diced
    5   scallions, finely chopped
    ½   cup dry-roasted pecans, finely chopped
    1   cup (or to taste) Italian Vinaigrette Dressing (see p. 296)

Cook quinoa for 10–15 minutes (see cooking instructions, page 288). Drain and let cool. Add peppers, scallions, pecans, and dressing. Stir and serve.

Hot Quinoa Cereal

    1   cup unsweetened almond or coconut milk
    ⅓   cup Quinoa Flakes (Ancient Harvest Quinoa)
        Dash of sea salt
        Frozen organic blueberries, handful
        Liquid stevia

Add quinoa flakes and salt to rapidly boiling milk. Return to boil and cook for 90 seconds, stirring frequently. Remove from heat and allow to cool (cereal will thicken slightly). Add stevia to taste and a handful of frozen blueberries—the heat of the cereal will defrost the blueberries.

Nutty Brown Rice

1   cup brown basmati rice; rinse well and
    soak for 20 minutes in water
1   tbsp grapeseed oil
½   cup raw pine nuts
2   tsp ground cumin
½   tsp ground cardamom
2   cups water for cooking
    Sea salt and pepper to taste

Rinse rice thoroughly. In a pan over low heat, combine grapeseed oil, uncooked basmati rice, cumin, and cardamom. Stir frequently for 5 minutes. Add 2 cups of water, sea salt, and pepper. Bring to a boil. Reduce flame, cover, and simmer for 10 minutes. In a separate pan, roast pine nuts over a low flame, stirring frequently until lightly browned. Turn off the flame under the rice and let the rice sit for another 10 minutes over the burner. Mix in pine nuts and serve.

Amaranth Tabouli

1   cup amaranth, uncooked
2½ cups water
1   cup parsley, chopped
½   cup scallions, chopped
2   tbsp fresh mint
½   cup lemon juice
¼   cup olive oil
2   garlic cloves, pressed

Rinse amaranth. Put 1 cup amaranth into a pot with 2½ cups of water and bring to a boil. Reduce heat, cover, and simmer for 20 minutes. Let cool. Place rest of ingredients into a mixing bowl, add amaranth, and toss together lightly. Chill for an hour or more to allow flavors to blend.

DESSERTS AND SNACKS

Pumpkin Pie

CRUST:*

- ½ cup arrowroot powder
- ¼ cup almond meal flour†
- ¾ cup amaranth flour
- ¼ tsp sea salt
- ½ tsp ground cinnamon
- 3 tbsp grapeseed oil
- 3–4 tbsp water

Preheat oven to 400°. Oil a 9-inch pie pan; set aside. Combine dry ingredients and blend well. Combine oil and 3 tablespoons water and blend with fork. Add all at once to flour. Stir only until a ball forms. If ball appears dry and crumbly, add a little more water, one teaspoon at a time, until ball hangs together. (Moisture content of flour varies.) Put the ball in the pie pan and use your palms to flatten it as much as possible. Use your thumbs and the knuckles of your fist to flatten it further and spread the crust as evenly as possibly to fit the pie pan. (The original recipe reads as follows, but it is nearly impossible to roll this crust: "Pat or roll crust to fit into pie pan. Dough tears easily, but mends easily using extra bits to patch.") Prick with fork. Bake 3 minutes in 400° oven. Remove from oven and set aside. Lower oven temperature to 350°.

PUMPKIN PIE FILLING:

- 2 cups pumpkin pulp‡
- 2 eggs
- ¾ cup Just Like Sugar (table-top style)

*The pie crust recipe is a slightly modified version of the recipe found on www.bobsredmill.com.

†You can buy this from Bob's Red Mill or make it yourself with a food processor, using blanched almonds.

‡Fresh pumpkin (baked or steamed) always tastes better than canned, so use that if you have the time to cook it yourself.

½ tsp sea salt
1 tsp ground ginger
1 tsp ground cinnamon
½ tsp ground cloves
1½ cups coconut milk*

Blend all ingredients together in a blender or food processor. Pour into pie crust and bake at 350° for 45–50 minutes or until knife inserted in the middle comes out clean.

Chocolate Ice Cream†
(requires ice cream maker)

⅔ cup cacao powder
1 cup Just Like Sugar (table-top style)
2 14-oz cans coconut milk*
¼ tsp stevia powder‡
1 tsp vanilla extract (alcohol-free)

Thoroughly mix all ingredients. Cover and refrigerate overnight. Pour the ice cream batter into your ice cream maker and follow your machine's directions.

Baked Cinnamon Apple

1 medium Granny Smith or pippin apple
1 tbsp butter, softened
1 tbsp cinnamon
   Pinch of nutmeg (optional)

Remove apple core to about ½ inch from the bottom of the apple. Make the hole about ¾- to 1-inch wide. Blend the cinnamon and butter and spoon it into cavity of apple. Place apple in a buttered baking pan with about ¼ inch of water and bake at 350° until tender. Sprinkle with nutmeg.

*Use Native Forest brand organic coconut milk because it has a better consistency; it can be purchased from www.vitacost.com.

†Avoid for first three months.

‡The batter isn't quite sweet enough with only the Just Like Sugar, and using this little bit of stevia will add the extra sweetness without thickening the batter by adding more Just Like Sugar.

Spicy Almonds, Walnuts, or Pecans

    1   cup raw almonds, walnuts, or pecans
        Few dashes of cayenne
  2–4   drops stevia liquid
    ¼   tsp sea salt

Stir all ingredients together. Spread on baking sheet and bake at 300° for 10 minutes.

Chocolate Nut Cookies*

    1   stick butter, softened
    ¼   tsp stevia powder
    1   egg
    ½   tsp vanilla extract (alcohol-free)
    ½   cup buckwheat flour
    ½   tsp sea salt
    ½   tsp baking soda
    1   cup almond flour
    ¼   cup raw pecans or walnuts, chopped
    ½   cup unsweetened cocoa powder

Mix together the first four ingredients in a bowl. Add remaining ingredients in order. Drop tablespoonfuls of batter onto a greased baking sheet and bake 10 minutes at 375°.

Tahini Toast

    1   slice bread (Sami's Millet & Flax Bread or Paleo Bread)
    1   tbsp raw tahini
        Pinch of cinnamon
        Pinch of powdered stevia or drop of liquid

Blend tahini, cinnamon, and stevia, and spread on toasted bread.

Chocolate Pudding*

    ⅓   cup raw organic cacao powder
    ½   cup Just Like Sugar (table-top version)
    1   tsp vanilla extract (alcohol-free)

*Avoid for first three months.

1   can (14 oz) coconut milk

In a medium mixing bowl, gently stir all ingredients together until the dry ingredients are thoroughly incorporated into the wet ingredients. Whisk with an electric whisk on high speed for 2 minutes. Cover and refrigerate overnight.

Kale Chips

Lacinato kale
Olive oil
Sea salt
Other spices, as desired

Cut or tear small pieces of kale and massage with olive oil, sea salt, and spices. Bake at 250° for 20 minutes. Stir and bake for another 20 minutes.

BEVERAGES

Raspberry Lemonade

¼   cup fresh raspberries
¾   cup freshly squeezed lemon juice
Lo Han Sweet (Jarrow) to sweeten

Mix in blender, adding water if needed, and serve over ice.

Hot or Cold Cocoa/Cacao Milk*

1   cup unsweetened almond milk (plain)
½   tsp vanilla extract (alcohol-free)
1   tsp raw cacao powder or unsweetened cocoa powder
Stevia or Lo Han Sweet to sweeten

Heat in a pan if you desire it hot.

Hibiscus Mint Cooler (sun tea)

2   quarts water
½   cup hibiscus flowers
½   cup chopped fresh mint leaves

*Avoid for first three months.

Put hibiscus flowers, mint leaves, and water in glass jar and set outside in direct sunlight to make sun tea. Bring inside after an hour or two. Strain, and chill in refrigerator; serve over ice.

Chai Latte

Decaffeinated chai tea (hot or cold)
Splash of unsweetened almond milk

Citrus Soda

Sparkling mineral water (Gerolsteiner)
Wedge of fresh lemon or lime
1 drop stevia liquid

Ginger Ale

¾ cup peeled and chopped ginger root
3½ cups water
2 tbsp vanilla extract (alcohol-free)
1 tbsp lemon extract (alcohol-free)
¾ tsp stevia powder
Sparkling mineral water (Gerolsteiner)

Rapidly boil ginger root in water for ten minutes. Strain and place liquid in a jar. Stir in vanilla, lemon, and stevia. Cool and store in the refrigerator. Add sparkling mineral water to desired concentration when serving.

Kale-Ginger Smoothie

5 leaves of Lacinato kale, center stem removed
2 tsp chopped fresh ginger
¼ cup parsley stems and leaves
½ green apple, chopped
Juice of ½ lemon, freshly squeezed
½ cup water
1 drop stevia liquid (optional)

Blend until smooth.

Vegetable Alkalizer Juice

   3 stalks celery
   ½ small carrot
   ½ apple, green (no seeds)
   ½ cucumber
 4–5 large handfuls of raw spinach, watercress, chard,
      dark green lettuces, black kale,* dandelion greens,
      cilantro *and/or* parsley
   1 clove peeled garlic *and/or* 1-inch slice of ginger (optional)

Place ingredients in a vegetable juice extractor. Drink juice immediately on an empty stomach either an hour before a meal or 2–3 hours after a meal. Makes 8 ounces of fresh-squeezed juice.

Lemon-Poppy Seed Shake

   2 oz coconut milk (not low-fat), almond milk, or hemp milk
      (unsweetened)
   8 oz purified water
   ¼ tsp natural lemon extract (alcohol-free)
   1 tsp poppy seeds
   1 tbsp flaxseed oil
   2 scoops of Vitol 100% Egg Protein powder† (vanilla)
   2 tbsp nut butter (almond or macadamia)

Put all ingredients into a blender and blend.

Blueberry Buckle Shake

 6–8 oz coconut milk (not low-fat), almond milk, or hemp milk
      (unsweetened)
      Handful of fresh or frozen blueberries
   1 tsp natural vanilla extract (alcohol-free)
10–15 drops stevia liquid
   1 tbsp flaxseed oil

---

*Limit to 2–3 times a week due to its goitrogenic effect.

†Vitol 100% Egg Protein contains bee pollen. Do not use this product if you are allergic to bees or to any other bee products.

2   scoops of Vitol 100% Egg Protein powder* (vanilla) or Living Harvest's Hemp Protein Powder
Handful of walnuts *or*
2   tbsp nut butter (almond or macadamia)
1   tsp cinnamon

Put all ingredients into a blender and blend.

Protein Smoothie

6–8   oz almond milk or hemp milk (unsweetened)
1   scoop protein powder: egg-white (Vitol*), hemp (Living Harvest), or brown rice
Handful of kale or spinach
1   tsp coconut oil *or* 1 tsp almond butter
½   green apple
Handful of blueberries
Pinch of cinnamon
Pinch of xylitol or stevia (optional)

Almond Milk

1   cup blanched almonds
4   cups water (less or more for desired consistency)
⅛   tsp sea salt
1   drop vanilla extract (optional, alcohol-free)
3–4   drops stevia (optional)

Put all ingredients into a blender and blend. Put in glass jar and refrigerate. Will store for 6 days.

Herbal Teas

There are various teas to choose from, including lavender, mint, rooibos, chamomile, oolong, etc. Add stevia, lo han, or xylitol to sweeten if desired.

*Vitol 100% Egg Protein contains bee pollen. Do not use this product if you are allergic to bees or to any other bee products.

WHEAT ALTERNATIVES

The following list gives you an idea of the many ways you can enjoy grains and grain substitutes without using wheat. All grains used should be whole grain and not refined or bleached.

ALTERNATIVE	AVAILABLE IN THE FORM OF
Almond	Flour, meal, almond butter
Amaranth	Cereal, flour
Buckwheat	Cereal, flour, noodles, whole groats
Chestnut	Flour
Coconut	Flour
Hazelnut	Flour
Kañiwa	Flour, whole grain
Kelp	Noodles
Legumes*	Flours (black bean, fava bean, garbanzo bean, mung bean, pinto bean, red and green lentil, white bean)
Millet	Flour, whole grain
Oat*	Bran, flour, meal
Quinoa	Cereal, flour, whole grain
Rice (brown)	Bread, crackers, tortillas, rice cakes, whole grain
Sorghum	Flour, whole grain
Teff	Flour, whole grain
White bean*	Flour
Wild rice	Flour, whole grain, rice cakes

*Avoid for first three months.

RECOMMENDED PRODUCTS

Many of the recipes in the Recipes section include ingredients that can usually be found in your local health food store. Buying some of these products and keeping them on hand will give you a head start and help make your daily food choices easier. If your store does not carry an item listed below, let them know you are a regular customer and ask them to special order it for you, or order it on the Internet directly from the company or affiliated sites that sell those products, such as www.amazon.com, www.vitacost.com, and www.iherb.com. You may also find other brands not listed here—just check the ingredients carefully to make sure they don't contain anything you shouldn't be eating on the candida-cure diet.

PRODUCT	BRAND NAME
Breads (yeast-, gluten-, dairy-, sugar-free)	
Brown or black rice tortillas	Food for Life
Millet & Flax Bread	Sami's Bakery
Paleo Bread* (almond or coconut)	Julian Bakery
Broths	
Organic Free Range Chicken Broth and Organic Vegetable Broth	Imagine
Butter	
Organic butter (unsalted)	Horizon
Organic Ghee (clarified butter)	Purity Farms
Goat's milk butter	Liberte
Cereals, Cold	
Qi'a Superfood – Chia, Buckwheat & Hemp Cereal (original flavor)	Nature's Path

*May cause bloating if you're sensitive to psyllium fiber.

Sprouted Cinnamon Cereal	Lydia's Organics
Simple Granola	Go Raw

Cereals, Hot

Amaranth, brown rice, oatmeal (gluten-free, after 3 months), teff	Bob's Red Mill
Brown Rice Cream	Erewhon
Cream of Buckwheat	Pocono
Quinoa Flakes	Ancient Harvest

Condiments

Coconut butter	Artisana
Garlic spreads (various flavors)	Majestic Garlic
Guacamole	Trader Joe's, 365 (Whole Foods)
Liquid aminos (unfermented soy sauce and soy-free seasoning)	Bragg, Coconut Secret
Mustard (with apple cider vinegar only)	Trader Joe's, 365 (Whole Foods), Eden Foods Organic Yellow/Brown Mustard
Organic Sea Kelp Delight Seasoning	Bragg
Pestos, dairy-free (spicy and mild)	Basiltops
Sea salt	Celtic Sea Salt, HimalaSalt, The Grain & Salt Society, Real Salt

Oils

Coconut, flaxseed, grapeseed, olive, sesame	Spectrum (or other brands that are cold-pressed or expeller-pressed)

Crackers

Brown Rice Cakes	Lundberg
Brown Rice Crackers	Hol-Grain Crackers
Flax crackers (raw crisps and crusts)	Mauk Family Farms
Flax and herb crackers (read ingredients)	Raw Makery
Various crackers (read ingredients)	Awesome Foods
Garden Herb, Pesto, Tomato Basil	Two Moms in the Raw
Pizza Flax Snax, Sunflower Flax Snax, Spicy Flax Snax, Simple Flax Snax	Go Raw

Drinks / Water

Apple Cider Vinegar All Natural Drink (Ginger Spice, Limeade, Sweet Stevia)	Bragg
Mineral water, sparkling	Gerolsteiner
Smart Water	Glaceau

Whole Grains and Flours

Brown rice	Lundberg
Buckwheat, millet, sorghum, & teff flours (organic)	Arrowhead Mills
Gluten-free grains, flours, wild rice	Bob's Red Mill
Pancake and Baking Mix, Almond Meal Flour, Sweet Rice Flour, and Brown Rice Flour	Authentic Foods
Pancake & Baking mix (buckwheat flax; contains small amounts of white rice flour, so use no more than once a week)	The Pure Pantry
Quinoa flour (organic)	Ancient Harvest
Waffle & Pancake Mix, Sugar-Free Muffin Mix, Perfect Flour Blend, Pizza Crust Mix	Namaste Foods

Meats, luncheon (high in sodium;
use small amounts)

Organic Roasted Turkey Breast, Herb Turkey Breast	Applegate Farms
Herbed-Roasted Turkey, Peppered Roasted Turkey, Naturally Oven-Roasted Turkey	Diestel
Oven-roasted turkey (no salt), uncured turkey salami	Whole Foods Market (in deli case)

Milk Substitutes (almond, hemp,
coconut—unsweetened*)

Almond milk, original and vanilla (unsweetened)	Blue Diamond Almond Breeze
Almond milk (organic), original and vanilla (unsweetened)	Pacific Natural Foods
Almond milk, coconut milk	365 (Whole Foods)
Almond & Cashew Cream (unsweetened; after 3 months)	MimicCreme
Hemp milk, original (unsweetened)	Tempt (Living Harvest)
Coconut milk (unsweetened)	So Delicious (Turtle Mountain)

Nuts & Seeds and Nut / Seed Butters

Almond Butter, Sunflower Seed Butter	MaraNatha
Coconut Butter	Artisana
Pumpkin Seed Butter, organic	Jarrow Formulas
Raw nuts, raw or dry-roasted almond butter, macadamia nut butter	Trader Joe's
Raw nuts and nut butters	Whole Foods
Sesame Tahini, organic	Arrowhead Mills

*Read the labels, as some of these companies make sweetened and unsweetened
varieties with the same name.

Tahini, organic	Once Again
Sprouted Pumpkin Seeds, Sunflower Seeds, Spicy Seed Mix, Simple Seed Mix	Go Raw

Pasta

Brown rice pasta	Lundberg, Trader Joe's, Tinkyada
Kelp noodles	Sea Tangle Noodle Company
Pasta Pisavera, Say Cheez, Taco Pasta	Namaste Foods
Penne, spaghetti, fettuccine, elbows, etc.	Rizopia Organic Brown Rice Pasta
Quinoa Pasta	Andean Dream
Taco Pasta	Namaste Foods

Protein Powders

100% Egg Protein (egg whites)	Vitol Products, Inc.*
Egg-white powder	NOW
Hemp Protein Powder, unsweetened	Tempt (Living Harvest)
Protein Energizer Vanilla Shake	Rainbow Light
Rice Protein, plain or vanilla	NutriBiotic
Amazing Meal Vanilla Chai Infusion	Amazing Meal

Salsa

African Hot Sauces	Brother Bru-Bru's
Habanero salsa	Frontera
Mild or hot salsa	Green Mountain Gringo
Mild or hot salsa	365 (Whole Foods)
Salsa	Tacupeto

*Vitol 100% Egg Protein contains bee pollen. Do not use this product if you are allergic to bees or to any other bee products.

Snacks / Treats

Chocolate Coconut Fudge and Green Apple Cinnamon bars	DNA Life Bars
Kale chips	Brad's Raw Foods, Alive & Radiant Foods
Nutty Nibbles (sugar-free varieties)	Nut Just a Cookie
Rox Chox (cacao with birch xylitol)	Rox Chox
Steve's Original Paleo Stix (grass-fed beef sticks)	Steve's PaleoGoods

Sweeteners

Chicory root (Just Like Sugar)	Just Like Sugar Inc.
Lo Han Sweet	Jarrow Formulas
Stevia, liquid and powdered (different flavors)	Sweet Leaf
SweetFiber (inulin fiber, lo han guo)	Purpose Foods
Xylitol powder (The Ultimate Sweetener)	Ultimate Life

Vinegar (always keep refrigerated)

Apple cider vinegar (raw and unfiltered)	Bragg, Spectrum
Rice vinegar (unseasoned, no sugar)	Marukan

SUPPLEMENT AND TREATMENT PROTOCOL

It's now time to look at the suggested supplement protocol for detoxifying and repairing your body. While I have provided specific instructions for taking the supplements, you will need to work in conjunction with your physician or health-care practitioner to make sure you are meeting your individual needs.

After you have completed the five-week nutritional makeover, start the full candida-cure diet and begin the supplement and anti-fungal protocol. **Those who are more progressed, i.e., not ambulatory, or are extremely sensitive to supplementation should skip to page 355 and begin by doing the Slow-Start Supplementation and Dietary Protocol.**

Here are some guidelines to follow as you embark on this treatment plan:

GENERAL GUIDELINES

- Check with your physician or health-care practitioner before taking any supplements to make sure he/she does not foresee a potential interaction with any pharmaceutical medications you are taking.

- Women who are pregnant or breastfeeding should only do the candida-cure diet and take a prenatal multivitamin-mineral supplement, vitamin D_3, pure-grade fish oil, and probiotics. Check with your health-care practitioner about the amounts to take. When you are finished breastfeeding, you may start implementing the detox and supplement regime.

- Do not start taking an antifungal if you are not moving your bowels at least once a day. This must be corrected before you start the antifungal. See the Supplementation for Additional Needs section, page 371, for supplements you can take for constipation.

317

- Purchase your supplements from reputable sources, such as a health practitioner, professional supplement companies, health food stores, or online vitamin warehouses such as vitacost.com, iherb.com, or amazon.com. In the Resources section, I have listed sources for purchasing all the supplements outlined in this section. The small amounts of soy in some of the products I recommend are acceptable and usually non-GMO. Supplements sold in drugstores and supermarkets often contain sugar, synthetic dyes, and fillers. Read labels to make sure they say "no added dyes, fillers, sugar, corn, or yeast."

- If you live outside the United States, look for comparable products with similar ingredients to the supplements I have suggested by going online and viewing the ingredient labels of these supplements.

- Periodically check my website, www.annboroch.com, for the latest updates on supplement changes that pertain to this section.

- If you experience an upset stomach when taking any of the supplements that are supposed to be taken on an empty stomach, you may take them after meals. If you experience diarrhea from any supplement, stop taking it for three days, and then try taking one pill once a day and see if you tolerate it. If you do, continue to build up slowly. If you do not, discontinue the supplement permanently.

- Remember to drink adequate amounts of water and herbal teas daily—one half of your body weight in ounces.

At first glance, you might feel overwhelmed by making new food choices and taking all of the supplements. To ease into the program, a week before beginning buy groceries and think about your different meal options, including what you can eat in restaurants while you're following the protocol. Order or purchase the recommended supplements for detoxifying and rebuilding your body (see Resources for vendors).

INSTRUCTIONS FOR
DIET, DETOX, AND SUPPLEMENTATION

FIRST MONTH: DAYS 1–30

Candida-Cure Diet

- You will need to follow this diet for a minimum of two years and possibly stay on it for your lifetime.

- Do not consume sugars, alcohol, legumes (for first three months), gluten grains, refined carbohydrates, corn, dairy products, fermented or yeast products, and trans fats.

- Follow the "Foods to Eat" and "Foods to Avoid" lists, beginning on page 251.

- After three months, you may add more foods into your diet, as noted in your "Foods to Eat" and "Foods to Avoid" lists.

Antifungal

Choose either an herbal or pharmaceutical antifungal based on your needs (see pages 113–116 for a more in-depth discussion of the pros and cons of the different options). Herbal antifungals can be taken for long periods of time, but it's important to rotate them every couple of months to make sure you're getting the maximum benefit of the different herbs and compounds in them.

Herbal antifungals are my recommended choice because they are easy to obtain and are also antimicrobial, which means the herbs address more than just yeast. They also target parasites, bacteria, and viruses, all of which are factors that contribute to autoimmune diseases.

Herbal antifungals:

- Candida abX (Quintessential Healing, Inc.)

- Candida Cleanse (Rainbow Light)

- Pau d'arco (tincture—Gaia Herbs; tea—Pacific Botanicals or Mountain Rose Herbs)

Prescription antifungals:

- Nystatin tablets (not liquid, because it contains sugar)
- Diflucan (for jump-start only)

How to Take Herbal Antifungal

If you are taking Candida abX, Candida Cleanse, or pau d'arco (in pill form), start with one pill a day for the first three days, and then work up slowly. After three days, take one pill twice daily for three days; and after six days, take one pill three times daily for three days. Take them one-half hour before a meal or with food if they upset your stomach. If you are using pau d'arco tincture or tea, start with forty drops of tincture or one cup of tea a day, and slowly increase every couple of days until you reach the recommended dose of 120 drops (approximately 1 teaspoon) of tincture or 3 cups of tea daily.

How to Take Pharmaceutical Antifungal

Nystatin: Start with one pill a day for the first three days, and then work up slowly. After three days, take one pill twice daily for three days; and after six days, take one pill three times daily for three days. Continue taking one pill three times a day. Take them one-half hour before a meal or with food if they upset your stomach. Nystatin can be taken for up to two years, but have your blood drawn twice a year to monitor your liver enzymes.

Diflucan: Those with symptoms of severe depression or anxiety may want to use Diflucan to jump-start the eradication of fungus. Diflucan should only be used at the beginning of your program, regardless of whether you will be taking an herbal antifungal or Nystatin. Ask your doctor to prescribe three 150 mg tablets. Take one tablet on the first day, take one tablet on day four, and take the last tablet on day seven. If you decide to use Diflucan for a longer period, have your doctor monitor your liver enzymes. After your jump-start of three Diflucan tablets, begin taking one of the herbal antifungals or Nystatin.

Notes:

- Remember that antifungals may make you feel worse before you feel better, so work the dosage up slowly to allow your system to keep up with the elimination of toxins. If you need more than three days to increase your dose, take more time—there is no rush.

- Do not start taking an antifungal if you are not moving your bowels at least once a day. This must be corrected before you start the antifungal. However, you may start the diet right away.

- If you are wheelchair-bound, bedridden, using a walker or cane, or are extremely sensitive to supplements, do not start with antifungals of any kind. Begin your program with the Slow-Start Supplementation and Dietary Protocol (see page 355).

Supplementation

The following supplements may be taken according to the recommendations given. When the usage instructions say to take a supplement "with food" or "after meals," they should be taken *right after* the meal. Another option is to take them *right before* your first bite of food. Some people prefer this because they feel too full and waterlogged when drinking so much liquid after they've eaten.

VITAMIN C (3,000–6,000 mg daily)

Vitamin C is needed to support adrenal function, nerve impulse transmission, healthy collagen synthesis, development of cartilage and bone, and integrity of capillaries and blood vessels. Buy a vitamin C that contains mineral ascorbates and/or bioflavonoids. Plain ascorbic acid crystals will irritate your stomach lining and intestines. Spread the dosage throughout the day because your body will absorb only so much at one time. The powder form is more bioavailable to your body than the pill form, but both work. Increase your dose of vitamin C slowly. Start with 1,000 mg daily and gradually increase the amount. If you experience diarrhea, cut back your dose by 1,000 mg. You can take the powder with or without food, but it's best to take the pills after a meal or snack.

Usage: Start with 1 pill (1,000 mg) daily and slowly work up to 1 pill 3 times daily or a higher dose if you desire (6,000 mg maximum).

Brands: QBC capsules (Solaray), Vitamin C 1000 mg capsules (Solaray), Quercetin + C capsules (Twin Labs), Ultra Potent-C Powder (Metagenics), Buffered Vitamin C Powder (Life Extension)

VITAMIN E (800–2,000 IU daily)

Vitamin E is important for protecting the body from free-radical damage and helping to decrease inflammation. When buying vitamin E, be sure the source is natural. Look for "d-tocopherol" on the label and not "dl-tocopherol," which is synthetic. Also, use an E vitamin that has mixed tocopherols and tocotrienols. Increase your dose slowly. Those who are ambulatory need to take 800 to 1,200 IU daily; those who are wheelchair-bound should start at 800 IU and work up to 2,000 IU.

Usage: 1 400 IU pill twice daily with food. If not ambulatory, take 2 pills twice daily (start with one 400 IU pill 2x/day for 2 weeks, and add 1,200 IU the next week to work up to 2,000 IU).

Brands: E Gems Elite (Carlson), familE (Jarrow Formulas)

Note: Do not take vitamin E if you're on blood thinning medication. If you will be having surgery, stop taking vitamin E two weeks before so your blood will clot properly. If you begin to noticeably bruise, reduce your dose.

VITAMIN D₃ (5,000–10,000 IU)

Vitamin D is needed for healthy neurological function, balancing the immune system, and maintaining bone density. Vitamin D deficiency is prevalent in people with MS. A high-carbohydrate diet can decrease vitamin D_3 absorption. The skin makes vitamin D when it comes into contact with direct sunlight, but most people with MS live far away from the equator and don't take in enough sun. Have blood work done once a year to check your vitamin D levels. Those with MS will want to be in the range of 60–80 ng/mL. If your levels do not increase when using pill form, switch to liquid drops.

Usage: 1 pill once or twice daily with food; or 3–5 drops on tongue once daily with food

Brands: Jarrow Formulas, Life Extension, Biotics Research (Bio-D-Mulsion Forte, 2,000 IU, liquid)

RepairVite (K-63, caramel flavor)

This herbal and amino acid supplement powder, containing L-glutamine, aloe vera, deglycerized licorice, flavonoids, phytochemicals, and antioxidants, has been formulated to restore and repair the intestinal tract and lining. It is essential to repair leaky gut to reduce the inflammatory process of MS. The plant sterols and ferulic acid esters in the supplement help support a healthy enteric nervous system with intestinal motility and secretion of digestive enzymes. This formula alleviates acid reflux, heartburn, ulcers, and brain fatigue, and stops sugar and carbohydrate cravings.

Usage: 1 scoop 1 time daily, upon arising, in 4–6 ounces of water. Take an additional scoop at bedtime if you have heartburn, reflux, numerous allergies, or intense gastrointestinal symptoms.

Brand: Apex Energetics

Gallbladder abX (work up slowly)

This herbal nutrient supplement stimulates bile secretion, eliminates toxins, enhances peristaltic action of the intestines, and improves fat digestion. If your gallbladder has been removed, this formula is even more essential to help with fat digestion.

Usage: 1 pill 3 times a day with food. Work up slowly by starting with 1 pill once a day for 3 days; then 1 pill twice a day for 3 days; then 1 pill 3 times a day.

Brand: Quintessential Healing, Inc.

Note: If diarrhea or stomach upset occurs, stop taking Gallbladder abX for 3 days and then start up again with 1 pill a day, slowly working back up to 3 pills a day. If diarrhea occurs again, stop taking altogether and replace with Liver abX (see page 330).

Gluco abX

This supplement contains a broad spectrum of vitamins, minerals, and pancreatic and adrenal glandulars to support improvement of blood-sugar levels and reduce sugar and carbohydrate cravings. Oxidative processes and free-radical damage are the major contributing factors to vascular and neurological damage in people with abnormally high blood-sugar levels. This formula is especially important for those who are hypoglycemic (low blood sugar) and/or have adrenal fatigue.

Usage: 1 pill 3 times a day with food

Brand: Quintessential Healing, Inc.

Mental Alertness

This herbal blend nutritionally supports oxygenation, circulation, and cognitive and brain function. It contains ginkgo biloba, gotu kola, rosemary, and eleuthero root.

Usage: 1 pill once a day without food, preferably upon arising

Brand: Gaia Herbs

Note: Do not take if you are on blood-thinning medication. If you will be having surgery, stop taking two weeks before so your blood will clot properly.

Red Clover Tea, organic (do not drink if you have ulcers, acid reflux, or grass allergies, or if you are on blood-thinning medication)

This herb cleanses your bloodstream, lymphatic system, liver, and kidneys.

Usage: Slowly work up to 3 or 4 cups daily by starting with 1 cup upon arising for 3 days, then 2 cups daily for 3 days, and so on. Do not drink after 4 p.m. during the first month because you might have difficulty sleeping. This is due to the tea's cleansing effect on the blood and lymphatic system. After a month, this should not be an issue. There is no caffeine in red clover herb.

Brands: Pacific Botanicals, Mountain Rose Herbs

Preparation: One heaping teaspoon of the loose herb makes one cup (8 ounces) of tea. To make 4 cups of the tea, bring one quart of filtered water to a boil, and turn off the heat. Add four teaspoons of the bulk herb to a large French press, add boiling water, let it steep for no more than fifteen minutes, and then slowly push the plunger down. Drink throughout the day. After brewing, you may add ice cubes to make iced tea. Make sure to consume whatever amount you make the same day or it will get moldy, even if stored in the refrigerator.

Note: If you need a substitute for red clover tea, drink 1–3 cups of dandelion root, chamomile, or peppermint tea daily instead. You can drink just one of these, alternate them, or mix and match.

MYNAX (chelated calcium, magnesium, and potassium EAP)

This essential mineral salt complex helps repair myelin and assists with the proper firing of nerve conduction. It may alleviate fatigue, tremors, spasms, headaches, and moodiness, and may also help with bladder and bowel control.

Usage: 2–3 pills twice daily with or without food. Take 3 pills twice daily if you are more symptomatic or progressed.

Brand: Koehler USA

METHYL B₁₂ (1,000 or 5,000 mcg)

This vitamin assists with myelin repair, supports the central nervous system, increases energy, and is important for the formation of red blood cells.

Usage: Put 1 pill under tongue and let dissolve; take upon arising on an empty stomach. Take 5,000 mcg if your energy is very low.

Brands: Methyl B-12 (1,000 or 5,000 mcg, Jarrow Formulas), No Shot Methylcobalamin B12 (1,000 or 5,000 mcg, Superior Source)

DIGESTIVE ENZYMES (optional)

You may not need digestive enzymes, because there are small amounts of them in Gallbladder abX and Gluco abX. However, if you are still burping, bloated, or feel as though food is not being digested after a couple of weeks on Gallbladder abX and Gluco abX, start taking digestive enzymes.

Digestive enzymes assist with the proper digestion, absorption, and assimilation of nutrients from your food. Because of poor diet and stress, many people do not digest and eliminate properly. If you have trouble digesting animal protein (burping and heartburn), buy an enzyme that contains pepsin and hydrochloric acid (HCl). If you have blood sugar imbalances (low or high), use a pancreatic enzyme that contains pancreatin, lipase, protease, and amylase. If you're vegetarian or have mild digestive complaints, use a plant-based digestive enzyme.

Usage: 1 pill 3 times a day with first bite of food

Brands: Super Digestaway (Solaray), Enzy-Gest (Priority One), Digest Gold (plant-based, Enzymedica)

IONIC FOOTBATH (optional, yet highly recommended)

As I discussed in Chapter 9, ionic footbaths are extremely beneficial in assisting the body eliminate toxins. I feel they are a necessity for keeping up with the overload of heavy metals, chemicals, and pollutants we continually take in from food, air, and water. This treatment is especially beneficial for those who are not ambulatory. You can either find a practitioner in your area who has an ionic spa or purchase a unit. The brand I recommend is the Ionic S.P.A. (see Resources).

Usage: One 15–20-minute footbath once a week. Doing this treatment more than once a week will leach too many minerals from the body.

Directions for the Ionic S.P.A.: Put enough warm tap water into your foot tub to cover the ionizer (white stick). When the white ionizer is covered with the warm water, connect the cord into the AC/DC converter and plug into an electrical outlet. If you see small bubbles coming out from the ionizer into the water, your unit is working properly. Make sure you put in enough water to cover the ionizer, but not too much, or the water may spill out when you put your feet in. To double the life of your ionizing unit, with every other use, flip the switch on the little black box attached to the ionizer rod cord.

Those with autoimmune disease, cancer, or chronic health conditions should soak their feet for only 15–20 minutes once a week. Those who are healthy and using this as a preventive treatment may soak their feet once every 10 days. After the footbath, wipe your feet with a clean towel, unplug your unit, and wash the white ionizer and foot tub with warm soapy water, and rinse well.

FIRST MONTH: Days 1–30 Supplement Schedule

Supplement	Upon Arising	Breakfast	Lunch	Dinner	Bedtime	After Meals	Empty Stomach
Antifungal[1] (herbal or Nystatin)	1		1 (½ hr. before meal)	1 (½ hr. before meal)			X
Vitamin C[2] 3,000–6,000 mg		1	1	1		X	X (powder)
Vitamin E[3] 800–2,000 IU		1		1		X	
Vitamin D$_3$[4] 5,000–10,000 IU		1	1 (optional)			X	
RepairVite[5]	1 scoop					X	
Gallbadder abX[6]		1	1	1		X	
Gluco abX		1	1	1		X	
Mental Alertness[7]	1						X
Red clover tea[8] 3–4 cups/day		2 cups	1–2 cups (afternoon)			X	X
Mynax[9]	2–3				2–3	X	X
Methyl B$_{12}$[10] 1,000 or 5000 mcg	1 under tongue						X

FIRST MONTH: Days 1–30 Supplement Schedule

Supplement	Upon Arising	Break-fast	Lunch	Dinner	Bedtime	After Meals	Empty Stomach
DigestiveEnzymes[11] **(optional)**		1	1	1			Take with first bite of food
Ionic footbath (optional)		One 15–20-minute footbath 1x/wk					

1. Take ½ hour before meals, or with meals if you forget or it upsets your stomach. Work up slowly to full dose: 1 pill/1 cup tea daily for 3 days; then 1 pill/1 cup tea 2x/day for 3 days; then 1 pill/1 cup tea 3x/day (full dose). For tincture, start with 40 drops and work up to 120 drops (approx. 1 teaspoon).

2. Start with 1 pill (1,000 mg) daily and slowly work up to 1 pill 3x/day or a higher dose if you desire (maximum dose 6,000 mg). Pills must be taken with food. Powder is best taken on an empty stomach.

3. Don't take if on blood thinners. If not ambulatory, start with (1) 400 IU pill 2x/day for 2 weeks, and add 1,200 IU the next week to work up to 2,000 IU. Reduce dosage if there is noticeable bruising. Stop taking 2 weeks before surgery.

4. May take 2 pills a day (10,000 IU). Take 10,000 IU if blood levels are below 30 ng/mL.

5. Mix in 4–6 oz. of water. Take additional scoop at bedtime if you have heartburn, reflux, numerous allergies, or intense gastrointestinal symptoms.

6. Work up slowly to full dose: 1 pill daily for 3 days; then 1 pill 2x/day for 3 days; then full dose—1 pill 3x/day. If diarrhea or stomach upset occurs, see note on page 324.

7. Take on an empty stomach. Do not take if on blood-thinners or aspirin. Stop taking two weeks before surgery.

8. Work up slowly to 3–4 cups daily: 1 cup/day for 3 days in the a.m.; then 2 cups daily for 3 days, and so on. Only steep tea for 15 minutes. May drink second/third/fourth cups in the afternoon, but do not drink after 4 p.m. for first month because it can keep you awake at night. Don't drink if you have ulcers, acid reflux, or grass allergies, or if you are on blood-thinning medication. As a substitute, drink 1–3 cups of dandelion root, chamomile, or peppermint tea daily.

9. Take 3 pills 2x/day if you are more symptomatic or progressed. May be taken with or without food.

10. Take 5,000 mcg if your energy is very low.

11. If you need these, take 1 pill 3 times a day with first bite of food (see page 326).

SECOND MONTH: DAYS 30–60

Candida-Cure Diet

Continue following the diet.

Antifungal

You can either continue taking the same antifungal you used during the first 30 days or rotate and use another herbal antifungal. Rotating herbal antifungals each month or every two months ensures you are getting the maximum benefit of different herbs and compounds to eliminate all unhealthy microbes, not just candida.

If you are taking Nystatin, continue taking it for six months to a year and then switch to herbal antifungals. Have your blood drawn twice a year to make sure your liver enzymes are normal.

Usage: 1 pill 3 times a day, ½ hour before a meal or with food if it upsets your stomach. If you have been drinking pau d'arco tea, drink 3 cups daily.

If you are switching to a different antifungal, work up slowly, starting with 1 pill for 3 days; then 1 pill twice daily for 3 days, and so on. If you are starting to use pau d'arco tincture or tea, take forty drops of tincture or one cup of tea a day, and slowly increase every couple of days until you reach the recommended dose of 120 drops (approx. 1 teaspoon) of tincture or 3 cups of tea daily.

Brands: Candida abX (Quintessential Healing, Inc.), Candida Cleanse (Rainbow Light), pau d'arco (tincture—Gaia Herbs; tea—Pacific Botanicals or Mountain Rose Herbs)

Supplementation

LIVER abX (work up slowly)
This formula contains key vitamin substrates and amino acids that support liver detoxification, as well as clinically validated herbs that support healthy detoxification reactions, hepatic (liver)

cell growth, and RNA synthesis. The goal of hepatic detoxification is to transform fat-soluble chemicals into less toxic water-soluble compounds so that they can be safely eliminated in urine, sweat, or bile. This supplement assists with two stages of the liver's detoxification process known as Phase I and Phase II.

Usage: 1 pill 3 times a day with food. Work up slowly by starting with 1 pill once a day for 3 days; then 1 pill twice a day for 3 days, and so on.

Brand: Quintessential Healing, Inc.

GLUCO abX or Adrenal abX

If you are continuing to struggle with hypoglycemia, have highs and lows of energy throughout the day, and/or still have sugar and carbohydrate cravings, continue on Gluco abX for one more month.

If these issues have resolved, switch to Adrenal abX. This powerful formula was designed to provide essential nutrients and co-factors that address chronic adrenal (parasympathetic) exhaustion resulting from an overworked mind and body. It is rich in digestive enzymes, several essential vitamins and minerals, and provides glandular support for the adrenals, pituitary, and spleen.

Usage: 1 pill 3 times a day with food. If you have trouble sleeping while on Adrenal abX, take 1 pill at breakfast and 1 pill at lunch, and skip the dinner dose.

Brand: Quintessential Healing, Inc.

Nrf2 Activator

Developed by Dr. David Perlmutter, this supplement is designed to activate the Nrf2 genetic pathway. This pathway regulates the body's production of glutathione and superoxide dismutase (SOD), both of which act as antioxidants. It also regulates the production of detoxification enzymes, including glutathione S-transferase, and down-regulates inflammatory factors such as NF-kB for a healthy response to inflammation. The formula contains broccoli seed extract, turmeric extract, black pepper extract, green tea leaf extract, and pterostilbene.

Usage: 1 pill once daily with food

Brand: Xymogen

Mental Alertness

Continue taking this supplement as you did during the first 30 days.

Usage: 1 pill once a day without food, preferably upon arising

Brand: Gaia Herbs

Note: Do not take if you are on blood-thinning medication. If you will be having surgery, stop taking two weeks before so your blood will clot properly.

Vitamin C (3,000–6,000 mg)

Continue taking this supplement during the second month of the program. Remember that if you experience diarrhea, cut back your dose by 1,000 mg. You can take the powder with or without food, but it's best to take pills after a meal or snack.

Usage: 1 pill 3 times daily or slowly work up to a higher dose if you desire (6,000 mg maximum)

Brands: QBC capsules (Solaray), Vitamin C 1000 mg capsules (Solaray), Quercetin + C capsules (Twin Labs), Ultra Potent-C Powder (Metagenics), Buffered Vitamin C Powder (Life Extension)

Omega-3 Liquid Fish Oil

Omega-3 fatty acids EPA and DHA are important for maintaining the fluidity and function of cell membranes, particularly those in the retina and brain. They also support the musculoskeletal and cardiovascular systems, immune health, and the structural integrity of neurological cells. I prefer fish oil in liquid form, as you can take higher amounts without having to swallow so many pills.

It is important to buy a brand that is free of harmful levels of PCBs. The brands I recommend below have disguised the fishy taste and have been tested for PCBs. If you must take gel capsules, take 2 pills (1,000 mg each) 2 times a day with meals.

Usage: 1 tablespoon once daily after a meal that contains some fat. Refrigerate after opening.

Brands: The Very Finest Fish Oil, Lemon (Carlson); High Concentrate EPA-DHA Liquid, Lemon (Metagenics); Ultimate Omega Liquid, Lemon (Nordic Naturals)

Note: Do not take fish oil if you are on blood-thinning medication. If you will be having surgery, stop taking the fish oil two weeks before so your blood will clot properly.

Evening Primrose Oil (1,300 mg)

This is an omega-6 essential fatty acid that is rich in gamma linoleic acid (GLA), which assists in repairing the myelin sheath, supporting a healthy inflammatory response, enhancing the strength of cell membranes, and balancing hormones.

Usage: 1 pill once daily with food

Brands: Evening Primrose 1300 (Jarrow Formulas), Evening Primrose Oil 1300 mg (Solgar)

Free-Form Amino Acid Complex (1,500–2,000 mg)

Amino acids are the building blocks of protein that are responsible for repairing and regenerating every cell, tissue, and organ in your body. They also assist the liver's detoxification process and are the precursors to neurotransmitters such as serotonin, GABA, dopamine, and acetylcholine.

Usage: 2 pills upon arising on an empty stomach; if it irritates your stomach, take after breakfast

Brands: AminoBlend (740 mg, Douglas Labs), Free Aminos (NutriCology/Allergy Research)

Vitamin E (800–2,000 IU)

Continue taking this supplement for second month of program.

Usage: 1 400 IU pill twice daily with food. If not ambulatory, take 2 pills twice daily or up to 2,000 IU.

Brands: E Gems Elite (Carlson), familE (Jarrow Formulas)

Notes: Do not take vitamin E if you're on blood thinning medication. If you will be having surgery, stop taking vitamin E two weeks before so your blood will clot properly. If you begin to noticeably bruise, reduce your dose.

METHYL B₁₂ (1,000 or 5,000 mcg)

Continue taking this supplement during second month of program.

Usage: Put 1 pill under tongue and let dissolve; take upon arising on an empty stomach. Take 5,000 mcg if energy is very low.

Brands: Methyl B-12 (1,000 or 5,000 mcg, Jarrow Formulas), No Shot Methylcobalamin B12 (1,000 or 5,000 mcg, Superior Source)

RED CLOVER TEA, ORGANIC (do not drink if you have ulcers, acid reflux, or grass allergies, or if on blood-thinning medication)

Continue drinking this tea during second month of the program.

Usage: 3–4 cups daily

Brands: Pacific Botanicals, Mountain Rose Herbs

Note: If you need a substitute for red clover tea, drink 1–3 cups of dandelion root, chamomile, or peppermint tea daily instead. You can drink just one of these, alternate them, or mix and match.

VITAMIN D₃ (5,000-10,000 IU)

Continue taking this supplement during second month of program.

Usage: 1 pill once to twice daily with food

Brands: Jarrow Formulas, Life Extension

MYNAX (chelated calcium, magnesium, and potassium EAP)

Continue taking this supplement during second month of program.

Usage: 2–3 pills twice daily with or without food. Take 3 pills twice daily if you are more symptomatic or progressed.

Brand: Koehler USA

TREVINOL PROFESSIONAL (work up slowly)

This is a blend of systemic and proteolytic enzymes, including serrapeptase, bromelain, nattokinase, protease, and papain, along with enzyme catalysts CoQ10, alpha-lipoic acid, quercetin, and magnesium. Systemic enzymes should be taken on an empty stomach to help remove circulating immune complexes, decrease inflammation and pain, improve blood flow, and reduce free radicals and fibrin.

Usage: 2 pills twice daily, either 30–45 minutes before a meal or 1½ hours after a meal. Work up slowly. Start with 1 pill twice daily for 5 days; then increase to 2 pills twice daily. If those times of day don't work for you, take them at another time on an empty stomach. One bottle might last more than one month, so continue to take until finished.

During exacerbations or times of extreme stress, work up to 3 pills twice daily: take 1 pill twice daily for 5 days, then 2 pills twice daily for 5 days, and then 3 pills twice daily. If you still do not experience relief from your MS symptoms, take 4 pills twice daily. Stay at 3 or 4 pills twice daily until you feel the exacerbation period has ended, and then reduce to 1 or 2 pills twice daily for another 2 months. You can take a course of enzymes for 1 to 3 months or take them for long-term maintenance at a dose of 1 pill twice daily.

Brand: Landis Revin

Other brands of enzymes: Vitalzym (World Nutrition), Wobenzym N (Garden of Life); see bottles for dosing instructions

Note: Because enzymes thin the blood and slow coagulation, do not take if you are pregnant; on blood thinning medication or aspirin; or if you have hemophilia, ulcers, gastritis, or extremely low blood pressure.

IONIC FOOTBATH (optional, yet highly recommended)

Continue doing one 15–20-minute footbath once a week.

SECOND MONTH: Days 30–60 Supplement Schedule

Supplement	Upon Arising	Break-fast	Lunch	Dinner	Bedtime	After Meals	Empty Stomach
Antifungal[1] (herbal or Nystatin)	1		1 (½ hr. before meal)	1 (½ hr. before meal)			X
Liver abX[2]		1	1	1		X	
Gluco abX or Adrenal abX[3]		1	1	1		X	
Nrf2 Activator		1				X	
Mental Alertness[4]	1						X
Vitamin C[5] 3,000–6,000 mg		1	1	1		X	X (powder)
Omega-3 Fish Oil[6]		1 tbsp				X	
Evening Primrose Oil 1,300 mg			1			X	
Free-Form Amino Acid Complex[7] 1,500–2,000 mg	2						X
Vitamin E[8] 800–2,000 IU		1		1		X	
Methyl B12[9] 1,000 or 5,000 mcg	1 under tongue						X
Red clover tea[10]	2 cups		1–2 cups			X	X

SECOND MONTH: Days 30–60 Supplement Schedule

Supplement	Upon Arising	Break-fast	Lunch	Dinner	Bedtime	After Meals	Empty Stomach
Vitamin D3[11] 5,000–10,000 IU		1	1 (optional)			X	
Mynax[12]	2–3				2–3	X	X
Trevinol Professional[13]	2				2		X
Ionic footbath (optional)	One 15–20-minute footbath 1x/wk						

1. Take ½ hour before meals, or with meals if you forget or it upsets your stomach. If switching to a new antifungal, work up slowly to full dose as you did for Days 1–30.

2. Work up slowly: 1 pill 1x/day for 3 days; then 1 pill 2x/day for 3 days; then 1 pill 3x/day.

3. Take either Gluco abX or Adrenal abX, not both. If you're still having hypoglycemia or sugar/carbohydrate cravings, stay on Gluco abX for one more month. If not, switch to Adrenal abX. Skip dinner dose of Adrenal abX if you have insomnia.

4. Take on an empty stomach. Do not take if on blood-thinners or aspirin. Stop taking two weeks before surgery.

5. Pills must be taken with food. Powder is best taken on an empty stomach.

6. Take after a meal that contains some fat. Refrigerate after opening.

7. If it irritates your stomach, take after breakfast.

8. Don't take if on blood thinners. If not ambulatory, take (2) 400 IU pills 2x/day or up to 2,000 IU. Reduce dosage if there is noticeable bruising; stop taking 2 weeks before surgery.

9. Take 5,000 mcg if your energy is very low.

10. Don't drink if you have ulcers, acid reflux, or grass allergies, or if you are on blood-thinning medication. As a substitute, drink 1–3 cups of dandelion root, chamomile, or peppermint tea daily.

11. May take 2 pills a day (10,000 IU). Take 10,000 if blood levels are below 30 ng/mL.

12. Take 3 pills 2x/day if you are more symptomatic or progressed.

13. Start with 1 pill 2x/day for 5 days; then increase to 2 pills 2x/day. Take either 30-45 minutes before a meal or 1–1½ hours after a meal. (For exacerbations, see p. 335.) Do not take if you're pregnant, on blood-thinning medication or aspirin, or if you have hemophilia, ulcers, gastritis, or extremely low blood pressure.

<u>THIRD MONTH: DAYS 60–90</u>

Candida-Cure Diet

Continue following the diet.

Antifungal

Rotate to a different herbal antifungal if you haven't already done so. If you are taking Nystatin, continue taking it for several months. Get blood drawn twice a year to make sure your liver enzymes are normal.

Usage: 1 pill 3 times a day, ½ hour before a meal or with food if it upsets your stomach. For pau d'arco tincture, take 120 drops (approx. 1 teaspoon); for the tea, drink 3 cups daily.

Brands: Candida abX (Quintessential Healing, Inc.), Candida Cleanse (Rainbow Light), pau d'arco (tincture—Gaia Herbs; tea—Pacific Botanicals or Mountain Rose Herbs)

Supplementation

LIVER ABX

Continue taking this supplement during third month of program.

Usage: 1 pill 3 times a day with food

Brand: Quintessential Healing, Inc.

ADRENAL ABX (optional)

If you are still experiencing exhaustion, fatigue, dizziness, and overall low vitality, continue taking Adrenal abX. It can be used up to 6 months if needed.

Usage: 1 pill twice a day with food

Brand: Quintessential Healing, Inc.

MULTIVITAMIN-MINERAL WITH HIGH-POTENCY B-COMPLEX

This complete daily formula is scientifically designed to deliver essential cellular energy and balance to vital systems and organs. It will help provide lifelong support to your brain, skin, eyes, and immune, circulatory, antioxidant, and energy systems.

Usage: 1 pill 3 times a day with food

Brand: Life Force Multiple, No Iron capsules (Source Naturals)

OMEGA-3 LIQUID FISH OIL

Usage: 1 tablespoon once daily after a meal that contains some fat. Refrigerate after opening. If you must take gel capsules, take 2 pills (1,000 mg each) 2 times a day with meals.

Brands: The Very Finest Fish Oil, Lemon (Carlson); High Concentrate EPA-DHA Liquid, Lemon (Metagenics); Ultimate Omega Liquid, Lemon (Nordic Naturals)

Note: Do not take fish oil if you are on blood-thinning medication. If you will be having surgery, stop taking the fish oil two weeks before so your blood will clot properly.

EVENING PRIMROSE OIL (1,300 mg)

Continue taking this supplement during third month of the program.

Usage: 1 pill once daily with food

Brands: Evening Primrose 1300 (Jarrow Formulas), Evening Primrose Oil 1300 mg (Solgar)

FREE-FORM AMINO ACID COMPLEX (1,500–2,000 mg)

Continue taking this supplement during third month of the program.

Usage: 2 pills upon arising on an empty stomach

Brands: AminoBlend (740 mg, Douglas Labs), Free Aminos (NutriCology/Allergy Research)

Nrf2 Activator

Continue taking this supplement during third month of the program.

Usage: 1 pill once daily with food

Brand: Xymogen

Vitamin C (3,000 mg)

Continue taking this supplement during the third month of the program. Remember that if you experience diarrhea, cut back your dose by 1,000 mg. You can take the powder with or without food, but it's best to take pills after a meal or snack.

Usage: 1 pill 3 times daily, or slowly work up to a higher dose if you desire (6,000 mg maximum)

Brands: QBC capsules (Solaray), Vitamin C 1000 mg capsules (Solaray), Quercetin + C capsules (Twin Labs), Ultra Potent-C Powder (Metagenics), Buffered Vitamin C Powder (Life Extension)

Vitamin E (800–2,000 IU)

Continue taking this supplement during third month of program.

Usage: 1 pill twice daily with food. If not ambulatory, stay at 2,000 IU.

Brands: E Gems Elite (Carlson), familE (Jarrow Formulas)

Notes: Do not take vitamin E if you're on blood-thinning medication. If you will be having surgery, stop taking vitamin E two weeks before so your blood will clot properly. If you begin to noticeably bruise, reduce your dose.

Methyl B₁₂ (1,000 mcg)

Continue taking this supplement during third month of program.

Usage: Put 1 pill under tongue and let dissolve; take upon arising on an empty stomach

Brands: Methyl B-12 (1,000 mcg, Jarrow Formulas), No Shot Methylcobalamin B12 (1,000 mcg, Superior Source)

MENTAL ALERTNESS

Continue taking this supplement during third month of program.

Usage: 1 pill once a day without food, preferably upon arising

Brand: Gaia Herbs

Note: Do not take if you are on blood-thinning medication. If you will be having surgery, stop taking two weeks before so your blood will clot properly.

CoQ10 + ALPHA LIPOIC ACID (ALA) + ACETYL L-CARNITINE (ALC) HCL

This combination formula features three antioxidant nutrients that have been shown to provide protection against free-radical damage and to promote cardiovascular and cognitive health. ALA enhances the antioxidant activity of vitamins C and E. ALC is a precursor to the important brain neurotransmitter acetylcholine, which contributes to the support of cognitive function and memory. This remedy has also been shown to be effective in maintaining blood pressure levels already within the normal range

Usage: 1 pill once daily with food

Brand: Vitacost CoQ10 + Alpha Lipoic Acid + Acetyl L-Carnitine HCl, 700 mg

RED CLOVER TEA, ORGANIC (do not drink if you have ulcers, acid reflux, or grass allergies, or if you are on blood- thinning medication).

Continue drinking tea during third month of program.

Usage: 3–4 cups daily

Brands: Pacific Botanicals, Mountain Rose Herbs

Note: If you need a substitute for red clover tea, drink 1–3 cups of dandelion root, chamomile, or peppermint tea daily instead. You can drink just one of these, alternate them, or mix and match.

VITAMIN D₃ (5,000-10,000 IU)
Continue taking this supplement during third month of program.

Usage: 1 pill 1 or 2 times daily with food

Brands: Jarrow Formulas, Life Extension.

MYNAX (chelated calcium, magnesium, potassium EAP)
Continue taking this supplement during third month of program.

Usage: 2–3 pills twice daily with or without food

Brand: Koehler USA

NANOGREENS

Even though you are eating vegetables in your diet, you need extra green superfoods. The ingredients in NanoGreens help reduce inflammation, support your immune function, improve mental acuity, increase energy, detoxify heavy metals and chemicals, and help you maintain strong bones.

Usage: 1 scoop mixed in 6–8 ounces of water, once daily upon arising on an empty stomach. Refrigerate after opening.

Brands: NanoGreens[10] (BioPharma Scientific)

IONIC FOOTBATH (optional, yet highly recommended)
Continue doing one 15–20-minute footbath once a week.

THIRD MONTH: Days 60–90 Supplement Schedule

Supplement	Upon Arising	Break-fast	Lunch	Dinner	Bedtime	After Meals	Empty Stomach
Antifungal[1] (herbal or Nystatin)	1		1 (½ hr. before meal)	1 (½ hr. before meal)			X
Liver abX		1	1	1		X	
Adrenal abX[2] (optional)		1	1			X	
Multivitamin-Mineral		1	1	1		X	
Omega-3 Fish Oil[3]		1 tbsp				X	
Evening Primrose Oil 1,300 mg			1			X	
Free-Form Amino Acid Complex[4] 1,500–2,000 mg	2						X
Nrf2 Activator		1				X	
Vitamin C[5] 3,000–6,000 mg		1	1	1		X	X
Vitamin E[6] 800–2,000 IU		1		1		X	
Methyl B12 1,000 mcg	1 under tongue						X
Mental Alertness[7]	1						X
CoQ10 + ALA + ALC HCl		1				X	

THIRD MONTH: Days 60–90 Supplement Schedule

Supplement	Upon Arising	Break-fast	Lunch	Dinner	Bedtime	After Meals	Empty Stomach
Red clover tea[8] 3–4 cups		2 cups	1–2 cups			X	X
Vitamin D₃[9] 5,000–10,000 IU		1	1 (optional)			X	
Mynax[10]	2–3				2–3	X	X
NanoGreens[11]	1 scoop						X
Ionic footbath (optional)							

One 15–20-minute footbath 1x/wk

1. Take ½ hour before meals, or with meals if you forget or it upsets your stomach. Rotate to a different herbal antifungal if you haven't already done so. Work up slowly, as you did with the first antifungal.

2. If you're still experiencing exhaustion, fatigue, dizziness, and low vitality, continue taking Adrenal abX. Can be used up to 6 months if needed.

3. Take after a meal that contains some fat. Refrigerate. Do not take if on blood-thinning medication; stop taking 2 weeks before having surgery.

4. If it irritates your stomach, take after breakfast.

5. Pills must be taken with food. Powder is best taken on an empty stomach.

6. Don't take if on blood thinners. If not ambulatory, stay at 2,000 IU. Reduce dosage if there is noticeable bruising. Stop taking 2 weeks before surgery.

7. Do not take if on blood-thinning medication or aspirin. If you will be having surgery, stop taking two weeks before.

8. Don't drink if you have ulcers, acid reflux, or grass allergies, or if you are on blood-thinning medication. As a substitute, drink 1–3 cups of dandelion root, chamomile, or peppermint tea daily.

9. May take 2 pills a day (10,000 IU). Take 10,000 IU if blood levels are below 30 ng/mL.

10. Take 3 pills 2x/day if you are more symptomatic or progressed.

11. Mix in 6–8 oz. of water.

FOURTH MONTH AND ONGOING

Candida-Cure Diet

Continue following the diet. You may eat the foods that were restricted during the first three months of the program, as long as they agree with your body.

Antifungal and Probiotic Rotation

Probiotics are supplements containing bacteria that help restore the natural balance of microorganisms (microflora) in the intestines. Repopulating the gut with beneficial bacteria reduces the growth of harmful bacteria and thereby helps the body to more efficiently perform its work of digestion, detoxification, elimination, and nutrient production and absorption.

If you have been taking herbal antifungals, during the fourth month you will stop taking them and take only probiotics. Beginning with the fifth month, you will rotate the antifungals and probiotics, taking the probiotics every third month. For example, for one month you will take Candida abX; the next month you will take Candida Cleanse; and the third month you will take only probiotics. Repeat this cycle for at least two years. If you keep your diet exceptionally clean—meaning free of alcohol, sugars, dairy, and gluten—you may reduce your dose of antifungals after two years, alternating them with probiotics.

If you have been taking Nystatin, during the fourth month you will add in a probiotic, but take it at a different time of day than the Nystatin. Keep taking probiotics and Nystatin until you finish your course of Nystatin. Then begin taking an herbal antifungal according to the instructions on pages 319–321, rotating it with other herbal antifungals every month or every other month. Once you have taken the antifungal for two months, you should rotate it with probiotics every third month, as explained above.

Antifungal Usage (when not rotating probiotics): 1 pill three 3 times a day, ½ hour before a meal or with food if it upsets your stomach. For pau d'arco tincture, take 120 drops (approx. 1 teaspoon) daily; for the tea, drink 3 cups daily.

Antifungal Brands: Candida abX (Quintessential Healing, Inc.), Candida Cleanse (Rainbow Light), pau d'arco (tincture—Gaia Herbs; tea—Pacific Botanicals or Mountain Rose Herbs)

Probiotic Usage: 1 pill twice daily, upon arising and at bedtime, on an empty stomach (requires refrigeration except as noted below)

Probiotic Brands: Flora 20-14 Ultra Strength (Innate Response Formulas), Ultimate Flora Adult Formula 15 billion (ReNew Life), Dr. Ohhira's Probiotics 12 Plus (Essential Formulas; does not require refrigeration), Primal Defense Ultra (Garden of Life; does not require refrigeration)

Supplementation

UltraImmune 9

This synergistic blend of 9 medicinal mushrooms is enhanced with natural absorption boosters and the best quality Coenzyme Q10 possible, ProCoQ10, to support immune function. Most major degenerative diseases are at least partially caused by the immune system's inability to correctly identify and destroy aberrant cells and invaders. Another benefit is that it restores glutathione (known as the "master antioxidant"), which scavenges free radicals and is the body's natural chelator. Dried mushroom extracts will not aggravate candida at this stage.

Usage: 1 pill 3 times a day with food. Work up slowly by starting with 1 pill once a day for 3 days, then 1 pill twice a day for 3 days, then 1 pill 3 times a day (full dose). Once you are asymptomatic and in remission for a few months, you can reduce to 1 pill once a day.

Brand: Gethealthyagain.com

Multivitamin-Mineral with High-Potency B-Complex

Continue taking this supplement during the fourth month of the program and ongoing for life.

Usage: 1 pill 3 times a day with food

Brand: Life Force Multiple, No Iron capsules (Source Naturals)

Omega-3 Liquid Fish Oil

Continue taking this supplement during the fourth month of the program and ongoing for life.

Usage: 1 tablespoon once daily after a meal that contains some fat. Refrigerate after opening. If you must take gel capsules, take 2 pills 2 times a day with meals.

Brands: The Very Finest Fish Oil, Lemon (Carlson), High Concentrate EPA-DHA Liquid, Lemon (Metagenics), Ultimate Omega Liquid, Lemon (Nordic Naturals)

Note: Do not take fish oil if you are on blood-thinning medication. If you will be having surgery, stop taking the fish oil two weeks before so your blood will clot properly.

Evening Primrose Oil (1,300 mg)

Continue taking this supplement during the fourth month of the program and ongoing for life.

Usage: 1 pill once daily with food

Brands: Evening Primrose 1300 (Jarrow Formulas), Evening Primrose Oil 1300 mg (Solgar)

Mental Alertness

Continue taking this supplement during the fourth month of the program and ongoing for life.

Usage: 1 pill once a day without food, preferably upon arising

Brand: Gaia Herbs

Note: Do not take if you are on blood-thinning medication. If you will be having surgery, stop taking two weeks before so your blood will clot properly.

Free-Form Amino Acid Complex (1,500–2,000 mg)

Continue taking this supplement during the fourth month of the program and ongoing for life.

Usage: 2 pills upon arising on an empty stomach

Brands: AminoBlend (740 mg, Douglas Labs), Free Aminos (NutriCology/Allergy Research)

Nrf2 Activator

Continue taking this supplement during the fourth month of the program and ongoing for life.

Usage: 1 pill once daily with food

Brand: Xymogen

Vitamin C (3,000 mg)

Continue taking this supplement during fourth month of program and ongoing for life. You may increase the amount if you choose.

Usage: 1 pill 3 times daily; increase the dosage if you wish to go beyond 3,000 mg (6,000 mg maximum)

Brands: QBC capsules (Solaray), Vitamin C 1000 mg capsules (Solaray), Quercetin + C capsules (Twin Labs), Ultra Potent-C Powder (Metagenics), Buffered Vitamin C Powder (Life Extension)

Vitamin E (800–1,600 IU)

Continue taking this supplement for the fourth month of the program and ongoing for life.

Usage: 1 400 IU pill twice daily with food. If not ambulatory, take 2 pills twice daily.

Notes: Do not take vitamin E if you're on blood-thinning medication. If you will be having surgery, stop taking vitamin E two weeks before so your blood will clot properly. If you begin to noticeably bruise, reduce your dose.

Methyl B₁₂ (1,000 mcg)

Continue taking this supplement for fourth month of program and ongoing for life.

Usage: Put 1 pill under tongue upon arising on an empty stomach.

Brands: Methyl B-12 (1,000 mcg, Jarrow Formulas), No Shot Methylcobalamin B12 (1,000 mcg, Superior Source)

Red Clover, Pau d'arco, Chamomile, Dandelion Root, Hibiscus, and Peppermint Teas, organic (do not drink red clover if you have ulcers, acid reflux, grass allergies, or are on blood-thinning medication)

In month four, it is good to rotate and mix and match the red clover, pau d'arco, chamomile, dandelion root, hibiscus, and peppermint teas. You can combine two or more together. To make 2 cups, steep two teaspoons of the herbs in 16 ounces of boiled water for 15 minutes.

Usage: 2 cups 4 times a week

Brand: Pacific Botanicals, Mountain Rose Herbs. There are several sources for organic chamomile and peppermint teas; check your health food store or online websites.

Vitamin D₃ (5,000 IU)

Continue taking this supplement for fourth month of program and ongoing for life.

Usage: 1 pill once daily with food

Brands: Jarrow Formulas, Life Extension

Mynax (chelated calcium, magnesium, potassium EAP)

Continue taking this supplement for fourth month of program and ongoing for life unless you are asymptomatic and in remission for a few months.

Usage: 2–3 pills twice daily with or without food

Brand: Koehler USA

CoQ10 + Alpha Lipoic Acid (ALA) + Acetyl L-Carnitine (ALC) HCl

Continue taking this supplement for fourth month of program and ongoing for life.

Usage: 1 pill once daily with food

Brand: Vitacost CoQ10 + Alpha Lipoic Acid + Acetyl L-Carnitine HCl, 700 mg

NanoGreens

Continue taking this for fourth month of program and ongoing for life.

Usage: 1 scoop mixed in 6–8 ounces of water, once daily upon arising on an empty stomach. Refrigerate after opening.

Brands: NanoGreens10 (BioPharma Scientific)

Ionic Footbath (optional yet highly recommended)

Continue doing one 15–20-minute footbath once a week or once every ten days if you are asymptomatic and in remission.

FOURTH MONTH: Days 90 and Ongoing Supplement Schedule

Supplement	Upon Arising	Break-fast	Lunch	Dinner	Bedtime	After Meals	Empty Stomach
Antifungal[1] (for those taking Nystatin only)	1		1 (½ hr. before meal)	1 (½ hr. before meal)			X
Probiotic[2]	1				1		X
UltraImmune 9[3]		1	1	1		X	
Multvitamin-Mineral		1	1	1		X	
Omega-3 Fish Oil[4]		1 tbsp				X	
Evening Primrose Oil 1,300 mg			1			X	
Mental Alertness[5]	1						X
Free Form Amino Acid Complex[6] 1,500–2,000 mg	2						X
Nrf2 Activator		1				X	
Vitamin C[7] 3,000–6,000 mg		1	1	1		X	X
Vitamin E[8] 800 IU		1		1		X	
Methyl B12 1,000 mcg	1 under tongue						X
Red clover, pau d'arco, dandelion root, hibiscus, mint & chamomile teas[9]		2 cups 4x/week				X	X

FOURTH MONTH: Days 90 and Ongoing Supplement Schedule

Supplement	Upon Arising	Break-fast	Lunch	Dinner	Bedtime	After Meals	Empty Stomach
Vitamin D$_3$ 5,000 IU		1				X	
Mynax[10]	2–3				2–3	X	X
CoQ10 + ALA + ALC HCl		1				X	
NanoGreens[11]	1 scoop						X
Ionic footbath (optional)	One 15–20-minute footbath 1x/wk						

1. If you've been taking herbal antifungals, you will stop taking them and take only probiotics for month four. (See p. 346 about rotating the two beginning in month five.) If you've been taking Nystatin, continue taking until you finish your 6-month to 1-year course, and then switch to an herbal antifungal. Take it ½ hour before meals, or with meals if you forget or it upsets your stomach. Rotate herbal antifungals (see p. 319). After taking for 2 months, rotate them with probiotics every third month (see p. 346).

2. If you're taking Nystatin, take both on an empty stomach at different times of the day. Check the label of your probiotics to see if they need to be refrigerated.

3. Work up slowly to full dose: 1 pill daily for 3 days; then 1 pill 2x/day for 3 days; then full dose. Once you are asymptomatic and in remission for a few months, you can reduce to 1 pill once a day.

4. Take after a meal that contains some fat. Refrigerate. Do not take if on blood-thinning medication. Stop 2 weeks before surgery.

5. Do not take if on blood-thinning medication or aspirin. If having surgery, stop taking two weeks before.

6. If it irritates your stomach, take after breakfast.

7. Pills must be taken with food. Powder is best taken on an empty stomach.

8. If not ambulatory, take (2) 400 IU pills 2x/day. Reduce dosage if there is noticeable bruising. Don't take if on blood thinners; stop taking 2 weeks before surgery.

9. Mix up and/or rotate combinations of the herbs. Drink throughout the day. Don't drink red clover if you have ulcers, acid reflux, or grass allergies, or are on blood-thinning medication.

10. Take ongoing for life unless you are asymptomatic and in remission for a few months

11. Mix in 6–8 oz. of water.

MOVING FORWARD

As I said in Chapter 8, curing candidiasis can take up to a minimum of two years or longer. Candida overgrowth can come back even more virulently if you go back to old habits of eating poorly. Even after you reach the end of the two-year period in which you have been clearing candida, you will need to follow a candida diet. Indulging in foods that contain sugar, dairy, yeast, and refined carbohydrates can easily reignite inflammation in the body. I highly advise avoiding alcohol permanently because of its neurotoxic effects on the central nervous system.

Once you are asymptomatic you might think it's okay to eat what you want again, but I would caution you. Remember that it's not just about feeling asymptomatic, but rather about putting MS to bed forever—and that means it's essential to eat a healthy diet permanently. If there is an occasional indulgence, don't beat yourself up, but get back on track.

As you add back into your diet the foods that were restricted for three months, pay attention to how you feel. If you notice intolerances and reactions after eating them, such as a rapid heartbeat or pulse (90 to 180 beats per minute), fatigue, itching internally or externally, hives, gas, bloating, headaches, or a stirring up of MS symptoms, eliminate those foods. This is a clear sign your body does not want them in your system.

In cases of MS, you will need to take at least a reduced dose of an herbal antifungal compound for the rest of your life. A reduced maintenance dose of Candida abX, Candida Cleanse, or pau d'arco is one pill twice daily, 40 drops of tincture twice daily, or one cup of tea twice daily. Rotate the antifungals with the probiotics as I explained above under "Antifungal and Probiotic Rotation" to make sure you're getting the full benefits of using them, and also rotate the different herbal antifungals. You will also need to increase your dosage during stressful periods, such as when traveling and during holidays.

SLOW-START SUPPLEMENT AND DIETARY PROTOCOL

The protocol outlined in this section is for those who are extremely sensitive to supplements, foods, and airborne elements, as well as for those whose MS is more progressed. If you are not ambulatory, are bedridden, wheelchair-bound, or using a walker or cane, you will need to follow this protocol for at least two months before switching to the "Days 1–30" protocol, beginning on page 319.

If you are unable to tolerate the supplements below, just stick to the candida-cure diet, and with time you can try incorporating some of them. The most important supplements to start with are RepairVite, Turmero Active, and Resvero Active.

GENERAL GUIDELINES

- Check with your physician or health-care practitioner before taking any supplements to make sure he/she does not foresee a potential interaction with any pharmaceutical medications you are taking.

- Women who are pregnant or breastfeeding should only do the candida-cure diet and take a prenatal multivitamin-mineral supplement, vitamin D₃, pure-grade fish oil, and probiotics. Check with your health-care practitioner about the amounts to take. When you are finished breastfeeding, you may start implementing the detox and supplement regime.

- Purchase your supplements from reputable sources, such as a health practitioner, professional supplement companies, health food stores, or online vitamin warehouses such as vitacost.com, iherb.com, or amazon.com. In the Resources section, I have listed sources for purchasing all the supplements outlined in this section. The small amounts of soy in some of the products I recommend are acceptable and usually non-GMO. Supplements sold in drugstores and supermarkets often contain sugar, synthetic dyes, and fillers. Read labels to make sure they say "no added dyes, fillers, sugar, corn, or yeast."

- If you live outside the United States, look for comparable products with similar ingredients to the supplements I have suggested by going online and viewing the ingredient labels of these supplements.

- Periodically check my website, www.annboroch.com, for the latest updates on supplement changes that pertain to this section.

- If you experience an upset stomach when taking any of the supplements that are supposed to be taken on an empty stomach, you may take them after meals. If you experience diarrhea from any supplement, stop taking it for three days, and then try taking one pill once a day and see if you tolerate it. If you do, continue to build up slowly. If you do not, discontinue the supplement permanently.

- Remember to drink adequate amounts of water and herbal teas daily—one half of your body weight in ounces).

INSTRUCTIONS FOR DIET AND SUPPLEMENTATION

SLOW-START: FIRST MONTH

Candida-Cure Diet

- You will need to follow this diet for a minimum of two years and possibly stay on it for your lifetime.

- Do not consume sugars, alcohol, gluten grains, refined carbohydrates, corn, dairy products, fermented or yeast products, legumes (for first three months), and trans fats.

- Follow the "Foods to Eat" and "Foods to Avoid" lists, beginning on page 251.

- After three months, you may add more foods into your diet, as noted in your "Foods to Eat" and "Foods to Avoid" lists.

Supplementation

The following supplements may be taken according to the recommendations given. When the usage instructions say to take a supplement "with food" or "after meals," they should be taken *right after* the meal. Another option is to take them *right before* your first bite of food. Some people prefer this because they feel too full and waterlogged when drinking so much liquid after they have eaten.

RepairVite

This herbal and amino acid supplement powder, containing L-glutamine, aloe vera, and deglycerized licorice, flavonoids, phytochemicals, and antioxidants, has been formulated to restore and repair the intestinal tract and lining. It is essential to repair leaky gut to reduce the inflammatory process of MS. The plant sterols and ferulic acid esters in the supplement help support a healthy enteric nervous system with intestinal motility and secretion of digestive enzymes. This formula alleviates acid reflux, heartburn, ulcers, and brain fatigue and stops sugar and carbohydrate cravings.

Usage: 1 scoop in 4–6 oz of water 2 times daily, upon arising and at bedtime, on an empty stomach. If you find you are sensitive to this product, work your way up to this dosage by starting with ¼ scoop once daily, and slowly increase the amount. If you continue on this product for more than one month, reduce the dosage by taking 1 scoop only once a day.

Brand: Apex Energetics

RESVERO ACTIVE

This is a concentrated source of resveratrol in liquid form that is self-administered with a syringe in order to provide the specific servings needed to support normal immune balance and healthy anti-inflammatory response mechanisms. Resveratrol is a substance found in the skin of grapes. The natural polyphenols in this supplement also support cardiovascular, intestinal, respiratory, and neurological health.

Usage: 5 ml (1 teaspoon) once to twice daily, with food. Refrigerate upon receiving.

Brand: Apex Energetics

TURMERO ACTIVE

This natural anti-inflammatory supplement is designed to provide a rich and concentrated source of curcumin (a substance in the herb turmeric) in liquid form. Syringe delivery provides the specific servings needed to support normal immune balance and healthy anti-inflammatory response mechanisms. It also provides polyphenol compounds that have been shown to support cardiovascular, intestinal, respiratory, and neurological health. Research has shown that curcumin is rich in antioxidants and helps support the immune system, the digestive system, the skeletal system, and liver detoxification processes.

Usage: 5 ml (1 teaspoon) once to twice daily, with food. Refrigerate upon receiving.

Brand: Apex Energetics

VITAMIN D₃ (6,000 IU)

Vitamin D, also known as the "sunshine vitamin," plays many important roles in the proper functioning of the body. Though classified as a vitamin, vitamin D is actually a key regulatory hormone for calcium and bone metabolism, and is essential for immune function and proper cell growth. Vitamin D is also needed for healthy neurological function. A high-carbohydrate diet can decrease vitamin D_3 absorption. Vitamin D deficiency is prevalent in people with MS. The skin makes vitamin D when it comes into contact with direct sunlight, but most people with MS live far away from the equator and don't take in enough sun. Have blood work done once a year to check your vitamin D levels. Those with MS will want to be in the range of 60–80 ng/mL.

Usage: 3 drops on tongue, with food

Brands: Life Extension (2,000 IU, liquid), Biotics Research (Bio-D-Mulsion Forte, 2,000 IU, liquid)

CELLULAR RECHARGE

This is an important remedy that needs to be taken before you undertake a detoxification program. Rich in homeopathic cell salts and oligo elements, it helps counter symptoms of free-radical damage and supports cellular metabolic processes for generation of more ATP and cellular energy. It is especially useful for people who are environmentally sensitive.

Usage: Slowly work up to 10 drops (in 2 oz. of water) 3 times a day on an empty stomach. Start with 3 drops once a day for 3 days; then increase to 3 drops twice a day for 3 days; then 7 drops twice a day for 3 days; and then 10 drops 3 times a day.

Brand: Apex Energetics

Note: If you are alcohol sensitive, put 30 drops in 6 oz. of water and leave out overnight so that the alcohol evaporates (this is for the full dose). Drink the next day in 3 equal parts of 2 oz. at a time.

PROBIOTICS

Probiotics are supplements containing bacteria that help restore the natural balance of microorganisms (microflora) in the intestines. Repopulating the gut with beneficial bacteria reduces the growth of harmful bacteria and thereby helps the body to more efficiently perform its work of digestion, detoxification, elimination, and nutrient production and absorption. The formulas listed below help to promote the growth of beneficial bacteria in both the small and large intestines.

Usage: 1 pill upon arising and 1 at bedtime, on an empty stomach

Brands: Flora 20-14 Ultra Strength (Innate Response Formulas), Ultimate Flora Adult Formula 15 billion (ReNew Life); both require refrigeration

METHYL B₁₂ (5,000 mcg)

This vitamin assists with myelin repair, supports the central nervous system, increases energy, and is important for the formation of red blood cells.

Usage: Put 1 pill under tongue and let dissolve; take upon arising, on an empty stomach.

Brands: Methyl B-12 (5,000 mcg, Jarrow Formulas), No Shot Methylcobalamin B₁₂ (5,000 mcg, Superior Source)

IONIC FOOTBATH (optional, yet highly recommended)

As I discussed in Chapter 9, the rate at which bodies are able to eliminate toxins can be slow, especially if you are not ambulatory, and ionic footbaths are extremely beneficial in assisting with the detoxification process. I feel they are a necessity for keeping up with the overload of heavy metals, chemicals, and pollutants we continually take in from food, air, and water. You can either find a practitioner in your area who has an ionic spa or purchase a unit. The brand I recommend is the Ionic S.P.A. (see Resources).

Usage: One 15-minute footbath once a week. Doing this treatment more than once a week will leach too many minerals from the body.

Directions for the Ionic S.P.A.: Put enough warm tap water into your foot tub to cover the ionizer (white stick). When the white ionizer is covered with the warm water, connect the cord into the

AC/DC converter and plug into an electrical outlet. If you see small bubbles coming out from the ionizer into the water, your unit is working properly. Make sure you put in enough water to cover the ionizer, but not too much, or the water may spill out when you put your feet in. To double the life of your ionizing unit, with every other use, flip the switch on the little black box attached to the ionizer rod cord.

Those with autoimmune disease, cancer, or chronic health conditions should soak their feet for only 15 minutes once a week. After the footbath, wipe your feet with a clean towel, unplug your unit, and wash the white ionizer and foot tub with warm soapy water, and rinse well.

ANGLE THERAPY

Those who are not ambulatory and/or use a cane need to do angle therapy each day to help stimulate circulation and move toxins out from the lower extremities. For five minutes twice daily, lie on a bed or any flat surface on which you can elevate your legs above your heart and support your feet against a wall or on a chair. Or you can have someone hold your legs up—they don't have to be high above your heart, just high enough so that blood flow is moving from your feet and legs toward your head. This mechanically moves stagnant blood from your lower extremities.

SLOW-START: First Month Supplement Schedule

Supplement	Upon Arising	Break-fast	Lunch	Dinner	Bedtime	After Meals	Empty Stomach
RepairVite[1]	1 scoop in 4–6 oz. water				1 scoop in 4–6 oz. water		X
Resvero Active[2]		1 tsp		1 tsp (optional)		X	
Turmero Active[3]		1 tsp		1 tsp (optional)		X	
Vitamin D₃ 6,000 IU		3 drops				X	
Cellular Recharge[4]	10 drops in 2 oz. water		10 drops in 2 oz. water		10 drops in 2 oz. water		X
Probiotic[5]	1				1		X
Methyl B₁₂ 5,000 mcg	1 under tongue						X
Ionic footbath (optional)	One 15-minute footbath 1x/week						
Angle therapy	5 minutes 2x/day						

1. If you are sensitive to this product, work your way up to full dosage by starting with ¼ scoop 1x/day, and slowly increase the amount. If you continue on this for more than one month, reduce the dosage by taking 1 scoop only once a day.

2. Refrigerate.

3. Refrigerate.

4. Work up slowly to 10 drops 3x/day. Start with 3 drops in 2 oz. water 1x/day for 3 days; then increase to 3 drops 2x/day for 3 days; then increase to 7 drops 2x/day for 3 days; and then 10 drops 3x/day. Take at least 15 minutes before eating. If you're alcohol sensitive, put 30 drops in 6 oz. of water and leave out overnight so that the alcohol evaporates (this is for the full dose). Drink the next day in 3 equal parts of 2 oz. at a time.

5. Flora 20-14 Ultra Strength or Ultimate Flora 15 billion. Refrigerate.

SLOW-START: SECOND MONTH

For some, it is best to continue following the First Month Slow-Start Protocol (above) for another month or longer, particularly if your disease is progressing rapidly or you are bedridden. However, if you are getting stronger and tolerating the supplements well, you may choose to follow the suggested supplementation outlined below for the second month.

Candida-Cure Diet

Continue following the diet.

Supplementation

GLUTATHIONE RECYCLER

This amino acid and herbal dietary supplement supports the synthesis and recycling of intracellular glutathione, the primary antioxidant produced in our bodies. In a healthy body, glutathione is naturally recycled; however, this process is impaired when the body is overloaded with toxins. The formula provides essential nutrients, cofactors, and substrates that have been shown to aid glutathione activity, thereby supporting the immune system and cellular detoxification, and helping the body to be less reactive to foods, chemicals, and other substances.

Usage: 1 pill 3 times a day with food. Work up slowly by starting with 1 pill once a day for 3 days; then 1 pill twice a day for 3 days; then 1 pill 3 times a day.

Brand: Apex Energetics

GENTLE DRAINAGE

This is a mild homeopathic remedy for the gentle support and drainage of the connective tissue and elimination organs. Homeopathic phytotherapeutics and sarcodes help clear elimination channels. This product provides the ideal support that these organs need before stronger-acting remedies are taken for a more complete detoxification.

Usage: Slowly work up to 10 drops (in 2 oz. of water) 3 times a day on an empty stomach. Start with 3 drops once a day for 3 days; then increase to 3 drops twice a day for 3 days; then 7 drops twice a day for 3 days; and then 10 drops 3 times a day.

Brand: Apex Energetics

Note: If you are alcohol sensitive, put 30 drops in 6 oz. of water and leave out overnight so that the alcohol evaporates (this is for the full dose). Drink the next day in 3 equal parts of 2 oz. at a time.

RESVERO ACTIVE

This is a concentrated source of resveratrol in liquid form that is self-administered with a syringe in order to provide the specific servings needed to support normal immune balance and healthy anti-inflammatory response mechanisms. Resveratrol is a substance found in the skin of grapes. The natural polyphenols in this supplement also support cardiovascular, intestinal, respiratory, and neurological health.

Usage: 5 ml (1 teaspoon) once to twice daily, with food. Refrigerate upon receiving.

Brand: Apex Energetics

TURMERO ACTIVE

This natural anti-inflammatory supplement is designed to provide a rich and concentrated source of curcumin (a substance in the herb turmeric) in liquid form. Syringe delivery provides the specific servings needed to support normal immune balance and healthy anti-inflammatory response mechanisms. Also provides polyphenol compounds that have been shown to support cardiovascular, intestinal, respiratory, and neurological health. Research has shown that curcumin is rich in antioxidants and helps support the immune system, the digestive system, the skeletal system, and liver detoxification processes.

Usage: 5 ml (1 teaspoon) once to twice daily, with food. Refrigerate upon receiving.

Brand: Apex Energetics

VITAMIN D₃ (6,000 IU)

Continue taking this supplement during second month of program.

Usage: 3 drops on tongue, with food.

Brands: Life Extension (2,000 IU, liquid) Biotics Research (Bio-D-Mulsion, 2,000 IU, liquid)

CELLULAR RECHARGE

Continue taking this supplement during second month of program.

Usage: Take 10 drops (in 2 oz. of water) 3 times a day, on an empty stomach. Take at least 15 minutes before eating.

Brand: Apex Energetics

Note: If you are alcohol sensitive, put 30 drops in 6 oz. of water and leave out overnight so that the alcohol evaporates (this is for the full dose). Drink the next day in 3 equal parts of 2 oz. at a time.

PROBIOTICS

Continue taking probiotics during second month of program.

Usage: 1 pill upon arising and 1 at bedtime, on an empty stomach

Brands: Flora 20-14 Ultra Strength (Innate Response Formulas), Ultimate Flora Adult Formula 15 billion (ReNew Life); both require refrigeration

METHYL B₁₂ (5,000 mcg)

Continue taking this supplement during second month of program.

Usage: Put 1 pill under tongue and let dissolve; take upon arising on an empty stomach.

Brands: Methyl B-12 (5,000 mcg, Jarrow Formulas), No Shot Methylcobalamin B12 (5,000 mcg, Superior Source)

IONIC FOOTBATH (optional, yet highly recommended)
Continue doing one 15-minute footbath once a week.

ANGLE THERAPY

Those who are not ambulatory and/or use a cane need to do angle therapy each day to help stimulate circulation and move toxins out from the lower extremities. For five minutes twice daily, lie on a bed or any flat surface on which you can elevate your legs above your heart and support your feet against a wall or on a chair. Or you can have someone hold your legs up—they don't have to be high above your heart, just high enough so that blood flow is moving from your feet and legs toward your head. This mechanically moves stagnant blood from your lower extremities.

SLOW-START: Second Month Supplement Schedule

Supplement	Upon Arising	Break-fast	Lunch	Dinner	Bedtime	After Meals	Empty Stomach
Glutathione Recycler[1]		1	1	1		X	
Gentle Drainage[2]	10 drops in 2 oz. water		10 drops in 2 oz. water		10 drops in 2 oz. water		X
Resvero Active[3]		1 tsp		1 tsp (optional)		X	
Turmero Active[4]		1 tsp		1 tsp (optional)		X	
Vitamin D$_3$ 6,000 IU		3 drops				X	
Cellular Recharge[5]	10 drops in 2 oz. water		10 drops in 2 oz. water		10 drops in 2 oz. water		X
Probiotic[6]					1		X
Methyl B$_{12}$ 5,000 mcg	1 under tongue						X
Ionic footbath (optional)	One 15-minute footbath 1x/week						
Angle therapy	5 minutes 2x/day						

1. Work up slowly to 1 pill 3x/day. Start with 1 pill 1x/day for 3 days; then increase to 1 pill 2x/day for 3 days; then increase to 1 pill 3x/day.

2. Work up slowly to 10 drops 3x/day. Start with 3 drops in 2 oz. water 1x/day for 3 days; then increase to 3 drops 2x/day for 3 days; then increase to 7 drops 2x/day for 3 days; and then 10 drops 3x/day. Take at least 15 minutes before eating. If you're alcohol sensitive, put 30 drops in 6 oz. of water and leave out overnight so that the alcohol evaporates (this is for the full dose). Drink the next day in 3 equal parts of 2 oz. at a time.

3. Refrigerate.

4. Refrigerate.

5. Take at least 15 minutes before eating. If you're alcohol sensitive, see instructions in #2 above.

6. Flora 20-14 Ultra Strength or Ultimate Flora 15 billion. Refrigerate.

<u>SLOW-START: THIRD MONTH</u>

If you have successfully completed the first and second months of the slow-start protocol and you are feeling stronger overall, you may move onto the "Days 1–30" protocol, beginning on page 319. If you do not feel stronger, stick with the second month protocol until you feel you can move on.

SUPPLEMENTATION FOR ADDITIONAL NEEDS

The supplements listed below are for those who have additional and/or stubborn symptoms that need to be addressed while following the supplementation protocol during the first four months and beyond. Add them into the list of your daily supplements as needed. Those on the Slow-Start protocol may take them as well, as long as they are tolerated.

Some of the categories below include a few products that produce the same effect. Do your own research and try out the products to find those that work best for you and are most readily available to purchase.

Elimination Problems
(constipation or diarrhea)

To easily move through the detoxification process and restore health, you must have a minimum of one bowel movement each day. This is vital both while following the protocol as well as for the rest of your life. If you are not moving your bowels daily, choose a formula that works best for you. The goal is to have full, normal bowel movements, not diarrhea, so adjust the dose until it is right for you.

FIBER OR POWDER

Fiber sweeps the linings of the colon to remove plaque buildup, helps eliminate excess cholesterol, and keeps the stools formed. For constipation, take ground flaxseed meal daily (keep refrigerated). For diarrhea, use a psyllium powder.

Usage: Mix 1 tablespoon of organic ground flaxseed meal into 8 ounces of water or a smoothie, or sprinkle it over vegetables.

Brands: Organic ground flaxseed meal (Bob's Red Mill, Spectrum), Psyllium Husk Powder (Source Naturals)

If the flaxseed meal does not help the constipation, use one of the brands listed below, which are combination formulas that include flax, pectin, and other ingredients.

Brands: Gentle Fiber powder (Jarrow Formulas), FiberSMART (ReNew Life)

Usage: Take one level tablespoon in ten ounces of water. After the first week, increase the dosage to two tablespoons if needed, and take one tablespoon in the morning and one in the evening.

MILD LAXATIVES

If fiber isn't enough to get you eliminating daily, add or replace with magnesium citrate, aloe vera juice, or the Ayurvedic combination triphala, all of which have a mild laxative effect. These products are good for those who skip eliminating for only one or two days.

Usage: For pills, start with 1 pill once a day after dinner. If you do not have a movement the next day, increase to 2 pills after dinner, and so on, until you eliminate daily. Find the right dose for solid movements, not diarrhea. For powder, start with ½ teaspoon in warm water one hour before bed. Increase the amount if necessary. For aloe vera juice, drink 2–4 oz. upon arising and at bedtime, on an empty stomach.

Brands: Triphala (Himalaya USA); Magnesium Citrate (Vitacost); Natural Calm powder, raspberry lemon flavor (Natural Vitality); Aloe Vera Juice, whole leaf (Lily of the Desert, George's)

STRONGER LAXATIVES

These formulas are for those with stubborn constipation who don't move their bowels for at least 3 days or longer.

Usage: Start with 1 pill once a day after dinner. If you do not have a movement the next day, increase to 2 pills after dinner, and so on, until you eliminate daily. Find the right dose for solid movements, not diarrhea.

Brands: Aloe 225 (Bio-Design); Aloe Lite (Bio-Design; not as strong as the Aloe 225); Christopher's Quick Colon Formula Part 1 (Dr. Christopher's), Naturalax 2, Naturalax 3, or Aloelax (Nature's Way)

Exacerbations

SYSTEMIC / PROTEOLYTIC ENZYMES

During a flare-up, make sure to reduce all stressors, be strict on the candida-cure diet, and incorporate systemic and proteolytic enzymes to reduce inflammation and infection in the body. Trevinol Professional is one of the most potent enzyme complexes to help reduce inflammation and dissolve plaque in the veins and arteries. If you can't get Trevinol Professional, you may try one of the other brands listed below.

Usage: Work up to 3–4 pills upon arising and 3–4 pills before bedtime, on an empty stomach. Start with 1 pill twice daily for 5 days, then 2 pills twice daily for 5 days, and then 3 pills twice daily. Increase to 4 pills twice daily if there's still no relief from your symptoms. If those times of day don't work for you, take them at another time on an empty stomach (30–45 minutes before a meal or 1½ hours after a meal).

Brands: Trevinol Professional (Landis Revin; preferred brand), Wobenzym (Garden of Life), Vitalzym (World Nutrition)

Note: Because enzymes thin the blood and slow coagulation, do not take if you are pregnant; on blood-thinning medication or aspirin; or have hemophilia, ulcers, gastritis, or extremely low blood pressure.

HONEY-ROSEMARY TEA COCKTAIL

Honey brings oxygen to your cells and is a tranquilizer that relieves spasticity, while rosemary opens up breathing passages and balances the nervous system. This cocktail is beneficial for attacks, spasticity, and extreme fatigue. You can use honey during an exacerbation because your body recognizes that it is being used for an emergency situation, and it won't feed the candida.

Usage: Place 1 teaspoon of rosemary sprigs and/or needles in 8 oz. of boiling water. Let it steep for 5 minutes and strain. Place 1 heaping teaspoon of raw, unfiltered orange honey under the tongue and let it dissolve slowly. Then drink the rosemary tea.

Note: Avoid honey if you are allergic to bees.

Cold / Flu / Sinus / Sore Throat Remedies

COLLOIDAL SILVER

This potent natural antibiotic is helpful for colds, flus, sinus infections, and sore throats, and to prevent you from getting sick when traveling on airplanes or visiting foreign countries.

Usage: To help prevent illness during changes of season or when traveling abroad, take 3–5 sprays or drops daily under the tongue. Take the same dosage one time before boarding an airplane. If you feel you are coming down with an infection, take 3–5 sprays or drops 2–3 times daily until you feel better. If you are already sick, take 3–5 sprays or drops 4–5 times a day until you are well. For sinus infections, buy the vertical spray bottle and take 3–5 sprays or drops 4–5 times a day.

Brand: Silver 100 (Invision International, silver100.com)

WELLNESS FORMULA

This herbal-vitamin combination helps support your immune system to quickly knock out colds, flus, sinus infections, and viruses, especially when taken at the onset of the illness.

Usage: As directed on bottle

Brand: Source Naturals

TEA MADE FROM PAU D'ARCO, FRESH SAGE LEAVES, FRESH BASIL LEAVES, AND FRESH THYME (3–4 sprigs)

Steep 2 teaspoons of the herbs in boiled water for 15 minutes and strain. These herbs help eliminate a variety of infections, including those caused by viruses, bacteria, funguses, and parasites.

CHRISTOPHER'S LUNG & BRONCHIAL

This formula helps with upper respiratory infections and health issues related to change of season.

Usage: 2 pills 3x/day with food

Brand: Dr. Christopher's

FIRST AID THROAT SPRAY WITH ZINC & GSE

Good for sore throats.

Usage: As directed on bottle

Brand: NutriBiotic

WELLNESS HERBAL THROAT SPRAY

Good for sore throats.

Usage: As directed on bottle

Brand: Source Naturals

ALLER-LEAF

This herbal blend supports upper respiratory health.

Usage: As directed on bottle

Brand: Gaia Herbs

QUERCETIN + NETTLES

This formula is designed to alleviate allergies and provides support during changes of season. Studies have shown that both substances have anti-inflammatory properties.

Usage: 2 pills once a day with food if allergies are continual. During times of change of season, increase to 2 pills twice daily with food.

Brand: Designs for Health

Urinary Tract Infections and
Bladder-Control Issues

D-MANNOSE WITH CRANACTIN

This simple sugar, which does not feed candida, gets rid of E. coli bacteria and helps to prevent and eliminate mild urinary tract infections.

Usage: As directed on bottle; may be used daily to prevent further urinary tract infections

Brands: Solaray

U.T. VIBRANCE

This herbal blend has been formulated to alleviate mild to moderate bladder and kidney infections.

Usage: As directed on bottle

Brand: Vibrant Health

BLADDER-CONTROL

This herbal-vitamin blend is designed to reduce bladder overactivity.

Usage: As directed on bottle

Brand: The Natural Bladder

BETTER WOMAN

This is a Chinese herbal blend formulated to help with bladder-control issues.

Usage: As directed on bottle

Brand: Interceuticals, Inc.

KIDNEY BLADDER FORMULA

This combination of herbs helps to eliminate kidney and bladder infections.

Usage: As directed on bottle

Brand: Nature's Way

Insomnia

Quality sleep is one of the most important factors in allowing the body to heal. If you are not getting into a deep sleep or are waking up during the night, try some of the suggested formulas below. Make sure your room is as dark as possible so that your body secretes an optimal amount of melatonin, a hormone produced by the pineal gland that has antioxidant effects and aids sleep. Also, quit working or playing on electronic devices at least one hour before bedtime, and power down any devices in your bedroom. It's best not to have a TV in your bedroom, but if you must watch TV to help you fall asleep, choose a channel that is positive, not the nightly news, which will pump fear-based negative messages into your subconscious mind.

ORGANIC CHAMOMILE TEA

Chamomile is an herb that can assist with mild insomnia.

Usage: Steep in boiled water for 20 minutes and drink one hour before bedtime.

Brands: Traditional Medicinals, Pacific Botanicals

CALMING

This is a very mild homeopathic blend designed to relieve insomnia and restlessness.

Usage: As directed on bottle

Brand: Heel/BHI

TRANQUIL SLEEP

This formula contains L-theanine, melatonin, and 5 HTP.

Usage: As directed on bottle

Brand: Natural Factors

Note: Do not take if you are currently on pharmaceutical medication for sleeping or seizures.

BENESOM

This vitamin-herbal blend of melatonin, casein tryptic hydrolysate, and passion flower supports restful sleep and relaxation.

Usage: 1 pill 1 hour before bedtime. Can increase to 2 pills if needed.

Brand: Metagenics

Note: Do not take if you are currently on pharmaceutical medication for sleeping or seizures.

MELATONIN

This hormone, produced by the pineal gland, regulates sleep/waking cycles.

Usage: As directed on bottle

Brands: Life Extension (1 mg), Jarrow Formulas (Melatonin Sustain)

Note: Do not take if you are currently on pharmaceutical medication for sleeping or seizures.

Anxiety / ADD / ADHD / OCD

GABATONE ACTIVE

This powerful blend, containing vitamins, minerals, lithium orotate, valerian root, passion flower, and L-theanine, has been formulated to support GABA production. Studies have shown that GABA insufficiency is linked to conditions such as anxiety, ADHD, obsessive thoughts, the inability to relax, and lack of concentration.

Usage: Start with 1 pill once a day upon arising, with or without food. Increase amount slowly to find the dose that relieves anxiety and keeps you focused and calm. If you take more than 1 pill a day, spread the dosage out throughout the day. Maximum dose is 2 pills 3 times a day.

Brand: Apex Energetics

Note: Do not take this supplement if you are on Xanax or any other anti-anxiety medication.

L-THEANINE (100 mg)

An amino acid derived from green tea extract, L-theanine increases dopamine and GABA neurotransmitters in the brain. This supplement is milder than Gabatone Active, but is also formulated for the purpose of reducing obsessive thoughts and anxiety and increasing concentration.

Usage: Start with 1 pill upon arising, with or without food. You might need to increase to 1 pill twice daily; if so, take the second dose in the afternoon.

Brands: Jarrow Formulas, Source Naturals

Note: Do not take this supplement if you are on Xanax or any other anti-anxiety medication.

NEUROCALM

This blend of GABA, B vitamins, phosphatidylserine, inositol, chamomile, and magnesium is formulated to help with stress, anxiety, and chronic pain.

Usage: 2 capsules 1–2 times daily with or without food

Brand: Designs for Health

Note: Do not take this supplement if you are on Xanax or any other anti-anxiety medication.

Depression

ST. JOHN'S WORT

This is an herbal supplement with antidepressant and antiviral properties.

Usage: As directed on bottle

Brands: Gaia Herbs, Source Naturals

Note: Do not take this supplement if you are on MAO inhibitors or SSRI medications.

Serotone Active

This herbal-vitamin blend of St. John's wort, SAMe, B vitamins, and 5 HTP was designed to assist with serotonin production.

Usage: Start with 1 pill after breakfast, lunch, and dinner. Increase or decrease dose until you achieve the desired results. The maximum dose is 2 pills 3 times daily, with food.

Brand: Apex Energetics

Note: Do not take this supplement if you are on MAO inhibitors or SSRI medications.

5-HTP (100 mg)

This is a precursor to serotonin that aids in the production of melatonin.

Usage: As directed on bottle

Brands: Jarrow Formulas, Source Naturals

Note: Do not take this supplement if you are on MAO inhibitors or SSRI medications.

Musculoskeletal Pain

Glucosamine, chondroitin, and MSM

Glucosamine, chondroitin, and MSM are foundational components for repairing and supporting joints, tendons, cartilage, and bone.

Usage: As directed on bottle

Brands: Glucosamine + Chondroitin + MSM (Jarrow Formulas); Glucosamine Chondroitin Complex with MSM (Source Naturals); Extra Strength Glucosamine Chondroitin MSM, shellfish-free (Solgar)

Note: Do not take these supplements if you are allergic to shellfish, except for the Solgar brand.

Weight-Gain and Anti-Wasting Remedies

If you are having trouble keeping weight on, here are some suggestions. With each meal, eat a small amount of gluten-free grains (specifically brown rice) from the "Foods to Eat" list. Eat more winter squashes, such as pumpkin, butternut, acorn, etc. Eat avocado and nuts and nut butters daily. Make a protein smoothie with the protein powder listed below, using unsweetened almond, coconut, or hemp milk. Add 1 tablespoon of raw coconut oil (melted) or 1 tablespoon of almond or macadamia nut butter, and banana (allowed during the first three months for those who need to gain weight).

THE TRUE WHEY

This protein powder is made from the milk of contented cows. They are grass fed and never subjected to growth hormone treatment, chemicals, pesticides, or genetically modified organisms (GMOs). This product is allowed for the purpose of weight gain only.

Usage: As directed on jar

Brand: Source Naturals

Spasticity / Neuropathy / Restless Leg Syndrome / Pain

CANNABIS (make into a tea)

Drinking cannabis tea made from cannabis buds is very effective for spasticity, neuropathy, pain, insomnia, anxiety, depression, and many other symptoms. You must obtain a medical marijuana card in your state or check laws in your country. Check with your local dispensary and discuss which blend is best for your symptoms. Some cannabis blends are stimulating and help those who need more energy during the day or want to increase their appetite. Other cannabis blends will reduce pain and spasticity. *Do not eat edibles from dispensaries because they contain sugars and trans fats.*

Usage: Take 1 teaspoon of cannabis herb (buds), break apart, and put into a tea ball strainer. Place in a mug and add 1 teaspoon of unsweetened coconut milk or organic heavy whipping cream (this form of dairy is allowed only when making cannabis tea) to absorb the cannabinoids from the herb. Add 8 ounces of boiled water and steep from 10–45 minutes. The length of time you steep it will determine its effect. Experiment with the timing to find the strength you need to alleviate your symptoms. Drinking the tea on an empty stomach will result in a less "buzzy" feeling than drinking it with food. If you don't want to make a tea, you can put 1 teaspoon of ground-up herb into 1 cup of raw almond butter and mix well. Eat 1 spoonful of the cannabis-almond-butter mixture once to twice daily or as needed.

If you live in California or Colorado, there are THC oils available that you rub into your gums or inside of your cheeks in small amounts. Statewide Collective in California specifically makes an oil for those with MS.

HONEY-ROSEMARY TEA COCKTAIL

Use this only during exacerbations and in cases of extreme spasticity or extreme fatigue. Honey brings oxygen to your cells and is a tranquilizer that relieves spasticity, while rosemary opens up breathing passages and balances the nervous system. You can use honey during an exacerbation because your body recognizes that it is being used for an emergency situation, and it won't feed the candida.

Usage: Place 1 teaspoon of rosemary sprigs and/or needles in 8 oz. of boiling water. Let it steep for 5 minutes and strain. Place 1 heaping teaspoon of raw, unfiltered orange honey under the tongue and let it dissolve slowly. Then drink the rosemary tea. Honey brings oxygen to your cells and is a tranquilizer that relieves spasticity, while rosemary opens up breathing passages and balances the nervous system.

Note: Avoid honey if you are allergic to bees.

NeuroCalm

This blend of GABA, B vitamins, phosphatidylserine, inositol, chamomile, and magnesium is formulated to help with stress, anxiety, and chronic pain.

Usage: 2 capsules 1–2 times daily with or without food

Brand: Designs for Health

Note: Do not take this supplement if you are on Xanax or any other anti-anxiety medication.

Cenitol

This powder combination of magnesium, inositol, and citric acid promotes healthy nerve tissue synthesis and nerve conduction. It also supports a healthy mood by serving as a secondary messenger for several neurotransmitters.

Usage: 1 scoop in water 1–3 times daily. This supplement may produce loose stools, so you might want to start with ½ scoop once daily and build up to a dosage that helps with spasticity or neuropathy.

Brand: Metagenics

Extreme Fatigue

Honey-Rosemary Tea Cocktail

Honey brings oxygen to your cells and is a tranquilizer that relieves spasticity, while rosemary opens up breathing passages and balances the nervous system. This cocktail is beneficial for exacerbations, extreme spasticity, and extreme fatigue. You can use honey during exacerbations because your body recognizes that it is being used for an emergency situation, and it won't feed the candida.

Usage: Place 1 teaspoon of rosemary sprigs and/or needles in 8 oz. of boiling water. Let it steep for 5 minutes and strain. Place 1 heaping teaspoon of raw, unfiltered orange honey under the tongue and let it dissolve slowly. Then drink the rosemary tea.

Note: Avoid honey if you are allergic to bees.

B₁₂ SHOTS (from your physician)

Take these weekly for the first four weeks, and then monthly. Once your energy increases, you can switch to taking sublingual vitamin B12.

ORGANIC GREEN TEA

Drink one cup of the caffeinated tea in the morning and in the afternoon.

ADRENAL HEALTH

This herbal formula contains rhodiola root, holy basil, ashwagandha, wild oats, and schizandra berry. When the body is stressed, your capacity to adapt is reduced, which can wreak havoc on the immune, nervous, and inflammatory pathways. Optimizing adrenal gland function is essential to combating stress. This formula is designed to provide nourishment to the adrenals, thereby enabling the body to adapt to stress in a healthy way and restoring vitality.

Usage: 1 capsule 2 times daily, right after breakfast and lunch

Brand: Gaia Herbs

NADH (10 mg)

NADH stands for nicotinamide adenine dinucleotide (NAD) plus hydrogen (H). It is a naturally occurring coenzyme formed by vitamin B_3 and is found in all living cells. NADH is required for synthesis of adenosine triphosphate (ATP), the energy molecule used to power cellular functions and fuel body systems.

Usage: Dissolve 1 tablet under tongue, upon arising

Brand: Source Naturals (10 mg, Peppermint Sublingual)

DHEA

DHEA (dehydroepiandrosterone) is a hormone produced in the body and secreted by the adrenal glands. It acts as a precursor to female and male sex hormones (estrogen and testosterone). In supplement form it is designed to relieve extreme adrenal exhaustion and support overall health.

Usage: One 5 mg tablet at breakfast. You can increase this dosage to 10 or 25 mg if needed.

Brands: Youthful You DHEA 5 mg (Enzymatic Therapy, available through Vitacost)

Note: Do not take DHEA for more than six months without getting your saliva values tested. Stop taking if you start to have acne, more facial hair growth (women), and more anger and irritability. Do not take if you have a history of cancer.

KOREAN GINSENG

Korean (hot) ginseng is a root that can help with extreme exhaustion and support greater vitality.

Usage: 1 or 2 pills a day, taken at breakfast and lunch

Brand: Korean Red Ginseng (Imperial Elixir)

Thyroid Support for Radiation Exposure and Heavy Metal Removal

TRI-KELP

This blend of sea cabbage, bull kelp, and palm kelp supplies minerals and iodine to support healthy thyroid function and offset the negative effects of radiation and heavy metal buildup in the body.

Usage: Take ½–1 teaspoon daily. Put it in a smoothie with Nano-Greens or sprinkle it on salad.

ENVIRONMENTAL CHECKLIST

❑ Install air purifiers in home and office.

❑ Install water-filtering system at home or buy bottled water that has been purified (reverse osmosis, structured matrix, or distilled).

❑ Eliminate any mold growth in house or apartment.

❑ Put plants in bedroom and around the house to filter the air (English ivy, spider plant, peace lily, bamboo palm, philodendron, rubber plants).

❑ Eliminate synthetic pesticides and fungicides used on plants and in the garden.

❑ Service air conditioning and replace filters yearly. Service heating ducts and change furnace filters yearly.

❑ Replace down and/or feather pillows and comforters with hypoallergenic pillows and comforters.

❑ Remove baskets and dried flowers because they collect a lot of dust.

❑ Install a carbon-filter showerhead.

❑ Eliminate deodorants containing aluminum zirconium and propylene glycol. Weleda makes healthier deodorants.

❑ Use natural body-care products without chemicals and preservatives (search vitacost.com and iherb.com).

❑ Use natural, nontoxic cleaning products.

❑ When talking on cell or cordless phones, use a hands-free headset (with plastic air tube) or a speaker phone, but do not use Bluetooth devices.

❑ Avoid using microwave ovens to reduce EMF exposure.

❑ Sleep with your head facing magnetic north, if possible, to offset EMF radiation.

❑ Take Tri-Kelp daily to support healthy thyroid function and offset the negative effects of radiation (see p. 385).

BREATHING TECHNIQUES

It's important to breathe deeply each day. Most people who are leading stressful lives breathe shallowly from the chest up. However, correct breathing involves the full expansion of the abdomen and chest, starting from the groin and moving the air up through the belly, through the ribs, and into the chest. Taking one to three minutes a couple of times a day to practice deep breathing will help remove toxins and stress, and put you back into your point of power, the now moment. Proper breathing is crucial for supporting a healthy immune system.

Deep-Breathing Technique

1. Inhale: With mouth closed (or open if you have sinus or breathing problems), inhale slowly, expanding your belly, then your rib cage, and then your chest, to a count of seven. Hold your breath for seven seconds. (If your abdominal area doesn't move, put your hands on your lower abdomen, at the level of your navel, to help train yourself to feel this area expand with the breath.) Don't give up on your first try. Keep practicing. Sometimes it's easier to get the belly to expand if you start by lying down flat on your back. After you learn this movement, you can adjust to deep breathing while sitting up.
2. Exhale: Open your mouth slightly, with lips pursed, and exhale slowly, making a sound as if you are blowing out a candle; and to the count of seven, let the air leave first from your belly, then from your rib cage, and finally from your chest.
3. Optional: Each time you inhale, visualize golden-white and pink light entering through the crown of your head and penetrating your body to heal every cell, tissue, and organ. On each exhale, release any physical imbalances, tension, stress, fear-based emotions, and negative thoughts by feeling and seeing them leave as black smoke through the soles of your feet.

Breath of Fire
(cleanses the blood and stimulates the brain)

1. With your mouth closed, breathe in and out as if you're blowing out a candle with your nose.
2. On the inhale, expand your stomach outward.
3. On the exhale, pull the stomach in.
4. Inhale and exhale vigorously and quickly for approximately thirty seconds, being mindful not to get light-headed or dizzy from overdoing it or standing up too quickly when done.
5. Slowly work up to three minutes as you practice this exercise over time.

Moon Breath
(relaxes the body's parasympathetic nervous system)

1. Make an "antenna" with the fingers of your right hand by pointing them straight up to the ceiling. With the right thumb of that hand, block your right nostril.
2. Take a long, deep inhale, hold for ten seconds, and exhale through the left nostril. Do this for thirty seconds.
3. Slowly work up to three minutes as you practice this exercise over time.

Sun Breath
(energizes the body's sympathetic nervous system)

1. Make an "antenna" with the fingers of your left hand by pointing them straight up to the ceiling. With the left thumb of that hand, block your left nostril.
2. Take a long, deep inhale, hold for ten seconds, and exhale through the right nostril. Do this for thirty seconds
3. Slowly work up to three minutes as you practice this exercise over time.

STRESS BUSTERS

In this section you will learn some techniques for releasing stress from body and mind. If you find any of the movements in the exercises too difficult, don't force yourself; just do what is comfortable for your body. Most of these take ten minutes or less to do, so be good to yourself and take any needed breaks.

Shower Release

1. Stand in your shower and let the warm water caress the crown of your head. Imagine violet-colored light showering down on you. Take a deep breath and mentally give yourself permission to release everything negative, stressful, and fear-based that you've been holding onto, including other people's negative energy.
2. When you exhale, see and feel all your stress and fear draining out of your body through your fingertips and the soles of your feet. Let it all go down the drain.
3. When finished letting go, imagine golden-white and pink light coming out of the showerhead and going into your head and throughout your body. The golden-white light represents universal healing energy, strength, and wisdom, and the pink light represents unconditional love.
4. Breathe in this light and let it replace what you have just let go of. Inhale and feel the light entering and healing every cell, tissue, and organ, and bringing in more oxygen, energy, strength, courage, and hope.

Shoulder Roll

This exercise will help you feel more oxygenated and relax your upper body.

1. Starting with your left shoulder, roll it forward, up, back, and down, as if making a small circle. Do this three times. Inhale each time you roll the shoulder up. Exhale as you roll it back down.
2. Do the same on the right side, making three small circles.
3. When done with both shoulders, inhale deeply, and as you exhale, sound the word *ha* with your mouth open.
4. Repeat this complete cycle two more times.
5. When done, stick out your tongue and make it flutter in between your lips. Do this a few times.

Cat-Cow Flexions

1. Find a firm but padded surface. Kneel and place the palms of your hands on it. With your mouth closed, inhale while letting your back sag toward the floor and gently raising your head and looking up toward the ceiling. Don't force the movement.
2. With your mouth closed, exhale while dropping your chin to your chest and rounding your back upward. Do this for one to three minutes, starting slowly and then building up speed.

Exercise

Take a walk. Breathe, look at the landscape, the flowers, the sky, and the trees. Notice the sensuous pleasures of Mother Earth. Swimming, tai chi, qi gong, yoga, and cycling are also excellent ways to relieve stress and increase circulation.

Yoga Stretches

This exercise opens up the lower back and is great for people who sit all day at work.

1. Stand and spread your legs shoulder-width apart. Bend over without locking your knees, and let your arms and hands drop until they touch the ground. Stay there for one minute, taking deep breaths.
2. Keeping feet shoulder-width apart, bend your knees, lower yourself into a squatting position, and breathe. Keep your heels on the ground.

Strengthening the Optic Nerves

Eye exercises are important to help heal the optic nerves, which are commonly affected in those who have MS because of their condition and also from the stress of sitting in front of a computer, laptop, or other devices. Spend five minutes once or twice daily doing the following eye rotation exercises. The key is to feel the stretch in the eye muscles with each step you do.

1. Sit comfortably in a chair and look straight ahead. Without moving your head look up toward the ceiling or as far up as your eyes will go. Then, without moving your head, move your eyes as far to the right as they will go, then down towards the floor, then as far to the left as they will go, and then straight ahead. Repeat this rotation one more time.
2. Do the same rotation in a counterclockwise motion. Look up toward the ceiling, then to the far left, then down toward the floor, then to the far right, and then straight ahead. Repeat the counterclockwise rotation one more time. You will be doing two sets of each rotation.
3. Next, move your eyes in circles as if you are moving them around the numbers of a clock. Do this two times in a clockwise direction, and then twice in a counterclockwise direction.

Hug a Tree

Wrap your arms around a tree, leaning your body from the waist up against the trunk. Feel the tree pulling out the stress through the bottom of your feet. Inhale and exhale slowly for sixty seconds, releasing tension and stress from your mind and body.

Self-Hypnosis
(takes ten minutes)

1. Lie down or sit comfortably in a chair. Focus on a spot on the wall or gaze at an object. Fixate on it until you feel your eyelids getting heavy.
2. Close your eyes.
3. Take five slow, deep breaths.
4. Give yourself permission to relax every muscle, nerve, and fiber in your body. Visualize golden-white and pink light coming down into the crown of your head and spreading out through your scalp, face, and jaw as you simultaneously relax each of the associated muscles.
5. Feel the wave of relaxation and light extend from behind your head down your neck, back, and buttocks, and down the backs of the thighs, knees, calves, and feet. Let all tension, stress, and negativity go. Then visualize and feel the light and relaxation move into the tops of your shoulders and down your arms to your fingertips, and then into your chest, abdominal, and pelvic regions. Then visualize and feel it move down the front of your thighs, knees, calves, ankles, feet, and toes.
6. Feel the relaxation and light permeating every cell, tissue, and organ. Breathe.
7. Allow your mind to still for five minutes. Let conscious thoughts just pass by like clouds in the sky.
8. Once you've been in a still point for five minutes, focus on your body. Inhale golden-white and pink light into your brain and spinal cord. See your myelin sheath as smooth and continuous. (To help with visualization, look online for images

of nerves with a healthy myelin sheath.) Visualize your entire nervous system functioning optimally. Feel and imagine yourself being completely coordinated, walking, and free of any numbness or spasticity. If you see or feel any dark spots or imbalances, draw in the golden-white and pink light to that area, and as you exhale see the imbalances moving out through your feet. Feel and imagine yourself as whole and balanced in every cell, organ, and tissue.

9. Take three deep breaths and slowly return your awareness to the room.

10. Open your eyes and notice the difference!

FEAR BUSTERS

Submitting to fear can paralyze you, while acknowledging fear and releasing it can free you to move forward in your life with greater joy and ease. Many of our fears are ghosts from the past, whose memories haunt us and make us feel miserable in the present. The key is to stay in the present moment, seeing and accepting "what is" right now, and responding from that place.

Basic Process for Dealing with Fear and Anxiety

There are three basic steps to dealing with fear and anxiety:

1. First and foremost, you need to be aware of when you are feeling fear and thinking fear-filled or anxious thoughts. Denial will only make you feel more paralyzed.
2. Second, talking out loud to yourself is a powerful action step for dispelling fear and anxiety. Words are powerful, and their vibration rate when spoken out loud is seven times more powerful than that of words spoken internally. So immediately acknowledge and identify your fear-filled or anxious thoughts and feelings. Speak to them out loud. If you're in a situation where you can't speak out loud, speak to yourself silently.
3. Third, after you've acknowledge your fear-filled or anxious thoughts and feelings, give yourself permission to release them, and then replace them with positive thoughts and feelings or neutral actions. For example, take a deep breath, drink some water, or refocus on the work or activity you are doing.

In Chapter 13 I suggested speaking to your fears and anxieties as if they were people. When you have a fearful thought about your condition, you might say something like: "Okay, I see you trying to sneak up on me again. I accept that I'm feeling fear about the numbness in my legs. I'm really afraid I won't be able to walk."

Let yourself feel these words deeply as you speak them, and then say: "I give myself permission to release these thoughts and feelings now." Then replace your fear-filled and anxious feeling or thought with something peaceful or positive. For instance, say: "I am safe. I am healthy and whole. I can walk and will continue to walk. My central nervous system is getting better every day." Or just take a short walk, take a deep breath, call a friend, or read a book.

While going through this process, you might also use these visualizations:

1. After you acknowledge your negative and fear-filled thoughts, blow them into a large balloon of whatever color you choose. Tie a knot, set it free, and as it drifts into space, see the balloon explode in white light. Visualize your fear-filled thoughts and feelings dissipating into space.

2. Visualize a radio dial in your mind's eye. Hear, see, and feel the volume of your fear at ten on the dial. Start turning the dial from ten to nine, to eight, to seven . . . and feel your fear or anxiety diminishing as you turn down the volume. Feel the fear disappearing and becoming mute as you visualize the dial reaching zero.

3. As you acknowledge fear-based or anxious emotions and thoughts that arise, imagine in your mind's eye that they are floating past you on a ticker tape, and ask them to pass on by. Say: "I see you. Just keep moving. I don't have time for you today."

Acknowledge the Root of Fear

Many of our fears are rooted in our childhood experiences, so it's important for you as an adult to take control over the fearful little child that still lives inside you (your inner child). Offer that one reassurance that he or she is now safe and protected by your adult self. You can say: "We've both had enough of these fears, and I'm tired of being jerked around, so let's let this pattern go and do something different. That was then, and this is now." Taking this type of positive action and reassuring your doubtful child can turn negative spirals into positive ones.

Panic Attacks

If you feel a panic attack coming on, exhale all the air from your diaphragm, and at the end of your exhale release the sound "huh" three times. This forces the panic out of your body through the breath. Follow with a slow, controlled inhale that expands your belly, ribs, and chest as the breath moves upward (do not breathe from your chest up). Repeat until you feel calmer.

Gabatone Active (Apex Energetics) is an excellent supplement to help alleviate anxiety, panic, OCD, and lack of focus. You can also rub or press the area just below your collarbone next to your rotator cuff. This area is an acupressure point that opens up your lungs so you can take the full breaths that will help calm you down.

Lack of oxygen can make you feel anxious, fearful, or "speedy." Avoid lazy breathing, and practice deep breathing as often as you can during the day.

In times of panic, try incorporating the Emotional Freedom Technique or use my abbreviated tapping technique (see page 182). With the fingertips of your right hand, tap the side of your left hand—the fleshy part right beneath the bottom of your pinkie finger—and speak your affirmation. If you have privacy, speak out loud while tapping and say, "Even though I am terrified, can't breathe, and feel out of control, I deeply and completely accept myself." Keep repeating and tapping on that point until you feel calmer. If you are in a public place, you can tap while saying the affirmations silently to yourself, and it will still have an effect.

After using any of the techniques above, go outside for a short walk if possible. Walking helps to alleviate anxiety.

Moving through Fear

Realize that you are bigger than your fears and anxieties. Step back, and look down on your fear or anxiety as if it were a mass that you're holding in your hand. Remind yourself that you're more than this energy, which is simply the product of your past childhood experiences or imagination and which has no basis in your current reality. Remind yourself of all the other challenges you've met and moved through successfully. Do everything you can to encourage yourself to find new ways of releasing fear and anxiety so that they no longer paralyze you.

Make Action a Habit

Take action each time fear or anxiety surfaces. Repetition is what creates habits, so stick with acknowledging and getting rid of fearful thoughts and feelings each time they arise. If you do, you'll soon stop having them because you will have retrained your subconscious mind with a new habit, or come to a place of neutrality in the face of situations that used to trigger emotionally charged fear-based thoughts and feelings. The key is to remain aware and take advantage of the wisdom you have gained from the lessons you have learned from your past experience.

SAMPLE AFFIRMATIONS

Remember when giving your affirmations to state them in the present tense and to be specific with your words so that whatever changes you are envisioning come to you in a comfortable way. A good way to do this is to qualify your affirmation or desire with words such as "easily and effortlessly" at the beginning or end of your sentence. You may do that where you feel it's appropriate in any of the affirmations below or in any that you create yourself.

- I love, accept, respect, trust, and honor myself and my body unconditionally.

- I am expanding in spirit, in health, and in purpose. I am essential. I am whole.

- Every cell, tissue, nerve, and organ in my body is whole and balanced.

- I am whole and complete in myself, my life, my work, my purpose.

- I energize only those thoughts that are positive and supportive.

- I am safe and secure in all spaces and places. I am guided and protected.

- I am worthy because I exist. I exist; therefore I am worthy.

- I am patient and tolerant.

- I am peaceful, happy, and grateful.

- I am trusting. I let go and let God.

- I am free of fear and anxiety. I am sound of mind.

- I am courageous and tenacious.

- I am confident and powerful. My central nervous system is whole, balanced, and working optimally.

- My muscles are balanced and strong.

- I am lovable. I am okay just the way I am.

- I am successful personally and professionally.

- I will give to myself what I wish to receive from others.

- I am mentally and emotionally balanced.

CHALLENGING
OUTDATED BELIEFS

(See Chapter Fourteen, "Your Spiritual Self")

To do these exercises, find a comfortable environment where you won't be disturbed.

My Beliefs about Health

Step One: Take as much time as you need to contemplate these questions and get to the root of your deep-seated beliefs:

- Do I believe I can heal myself of a disease?
- Do I believe MS is curable or can be put into permanent remission?
- Do I believe I have the right to live a healthy life?
- Do I believe health is within my reach?
- Do I believe health is a choice?
- Do I believe I have the courage and strength to get well?

Step Two: For the following questions, write on a piece of paper any reflections that come to you about how these beliefs are currently impacting your life.

1. Do my present beliefs make me happy? If not, how are they contributing to my unhappiness?
2. Do these beliefs ring true to me at this time? If not, why not?
3. Do these beliefs keep me inflexible? If so, in what way?
4. Are these beliefs hand-me-downs that I received from someone else when I didn't consciously realize I had the power to choose my own beliefs (for example, when I was a child)? If so, from whom did they come?
5. Do these beliefs benefit my life, others' lives, and my world as a whole? If not, in what way are they detrimental?

Step Three: On a separate piece of paper, write out your new beliefs about health. At the top of the page write: "I now choose to believe . . ."

Step Four: Affirm these new beliefs every day with conviction and emotion. Think and act as if these new beliefs are true. Feel them, breathe them, affirm them by speaking them out loud, and mirror them until they truly become yours.

My Beliefs about Myself

Step One: Take as much time as you need to contemplate these questions and get to the root of your deep-seated beliefs:

- Do I believe I am worth my existence?
- Do I believe my worth is based on whether others love and validate me?
- Do I believe I am not good enough?
- Do I believe loving myself unconditionally is a key ingredient to health?
- Do I believe I have a purpose and can make a difference in this world?
- Do I believe that being good enough means being perfect?

Step Two: For the following questions, write on a piece of paper any reflections that come to you about how these beliefs are currently impacting your life.

1. Do my present beliefs make me happy? If not, how are they contributing to my unhappiness?
2. Do these beliefs ring true to me at this time? If not, why not?
3. Do these beliefs keep me inflexible? If so, in what way?
4. Are these beliefs hand-me-downs that I received from someone else when I didn't consciously realize I had the power to choose my own beliefs (for example, when I was a child)? If so, from whom did they come?
5. Do these beliefs benefit my life, others' lives, and my world as a whole? If not, in what way are they detrimental?

Step Three: On a separate piece of paper, write out your new beliefs about yourself. At the top of the page write: "I now choose to believe. . ."

Step Four: Affirm these new beliefs every day with conviction and emotion. Think and act as if these new beliefs are true. Feel them, breathe them, affirm them by speaking them out loud, and mirror them until they truly become yours.

My Beliefs about Love

Step One: Take as much time as you need to contemplate these questions and get to the root of your deep-seated beliefs:

- Do I believe I am worthy of being loved?
- Do I believe I can attract my equal?
- Do I believe my value depends on others' acceptance of me?
- Do I believe I can give and receive love?
- Do I believe sickness is a way of getting love and attention?

Step Two: For the following questions, write on a piece of paper any reflections that come to you about how these beliefs are currently impacting your life.

1. Do my present beliefs make me happy? If not, how are they contributing to my unhappiness?
2. Do these beliefs ring true to me at this time? If not, why not?
3. Do these beliefs keep me inflexible? If so, in what way?
4. Are these beliefs hand-me-downs that I received from someone else when I didn't consciously realize I had the power to choose my own beliefs (for example, when I was a child)? If so, from whom did they come?
5. Do these beliefs benefit my life, others' lives, and my world as a whole? If not, in what way are they detrimental?

Step Three: On a separate piece of paper, write out your new beliefs about love. At the top of the page write: "I now choose to believe . . ."

Step Four: Affirm these new beliefs every day with conviction and emotion. Think and act as if these new beliefs are true. Feel them, breathe them, affirm them by speaking them out loud, and mirror them until they truly become yours.

My Beliefs about Abundance

Step One: Take as much time as you need to contemplate these questions and get to the root of your deep-seated beliefs:

- Do I believe money defines my worth?
- Do I believe I am lacking because I don't have wealth or possessions?
- Do I believe being sick gives me an excuse not to succeed?
- Do I believe I deserve abundance, prosperity, and health?

Step Two: For the following questions, write on a piece of paper any reflections that come to you about how these beliefs are currently impacting your life.

1. Do my present beliefs make me happy? If not, how are they contributing to my unhappiness?
2. Do these beliefs ring true to me at this time? If not, why not?
3. Do these beliefs keep me inflexible? If so, in what way?
4. Are these beliefs hand-me-downs that I received from someone else when I didn't consciously realize I had the power to choose my own beliefs (for example, when I was a child)? If so, from whom did they come?
5. Do these beliefs benefit my life, others' lives, and my world as a whole? If not, in what way are they detrimental?

Step Three: On a separate piece of paper, write out your new beliefs about abundance. At the top of the page write: "I now choose to believe . . ."

Step Four: Affirm these new beliefs every day with conviction and emotion. Think and act as if these new beliefs are true. Feel them, breathe them, affirm them by speaking them out loud, and mirror them until they truly become yours.

My Beliefs about Success

Step One: Take as much time as you need to contemplate these questions and get to the root of your deep-seated beliefs:

- Do I believe I have what it takes to succeed?
- Do I believe being sick excuses from having to take risks and to move past challenges?
- Do I believe something always goes wrong and prevents me from succeeding?
- Do I believe in the fear of failure and/or the fear of success?
- Do I believe I have to struggle in life and that everything happens the hard way?

Step Two: For the following questions, write on a piece of paper any reflections that come to you about how these beliefs are currently impacting your life.

1. Do my present beliefs make me happy? If not, how are they contributing to my unhappiness?
2. Do these beliefs ring true to me at this time? If not, why not?
3. Do these beliefs keep me inflexible? If so, in what way?
4. Are these beliefs hand-me-downs that I received from someone else when I didn't consciously realize I had the power to choose my own beliefs (for example, when I was a child)? If so, from whom did they come?
5. Do these beliefs benefit my life, others' lives, and my world as a whole? If not, in what way are they detrimental?

Step Three: On a separate piece of paper, write out your new beliefs about success. At the top of the page write: "I now choose to believe . . ."

Step Four: Affirm these new beliefs every day with conviction and emotion. Think and act as if these new beliefs are true. Feel them, breathe them, affirm them by speaking them out loud, and mirror them until they truly become yours.

My Beliefs about Spirituality

Step One: Take as much time as you need to contemplate these questions and get to the root of your deep-seated beliefs:

- Do I believe in hope?
- Do I believe I can create my own reality?
- Do I believe I have a purpose in this world?
- Do I believe in God or a universal energy?
- Do I believe thoughts create energy?
- Do I believe fear-based emotions can weaken my immune system?

Step Two: For the following questions, write on a piece of paper any reflections that come to you about how these beliefs are currently impacting your life.

1. Do my present beliefs make me happy? If not, how are they contributing to my unhappiness?
2. Do these beliefs ring true to me at this time? If not, why not?
3. Do these beliefs keep me inflexible? If so, in what way?
4. Are these beliefs hand-me-downs that I received from someone else when I didn't consciously realize I had the power to choose my own beliefs (for example, when I was a child)? If so, from whom did they come?
5. Do these beliefs benefit my life, others' lives, and my world as a whole? If not, in what way are they detrimental?

Step Three: On a separate piece of paper, write out your new beliefs about spirituality. At the top of the page write: "I now choose to believe . . ."

Step Four: Affirm these new beliefs every day with conviction and emotion. Think and act as if these new beliefs are true. Feel them, breathe them, affirm them by speaking them out loud, and mirror them until they truly become yours.

WEEKLY OVERALL PROGRESS CHART (tracking your treatment plan)

	Mon	Tues	Wed	Thurs	Fri	Sat	Sun	Total
I ate a healthy diet.								
I did yoga, exercise, or physical therapy.								
I did breathing exercises.								
I maintained my schedule of supplements.								
I drank my quota of water and herbal teas.								
I did my dry skin brushing.								
I got enough sleep.								
I spent at least 15 minutes outdoors or in sunlight.								
I wrote in my journal.								
I spoke affirmations.								
I laughed and smiled.								
I meditated, did visualizations, or focused on positive thoughts.								

WEEKLY OVERALL PROGRESS CHART (continued)

	Mon	Tues	Wed	Thurs	Fri	Sat	Sun	Total
I released fear-based emotions and forgave myself.								
I read something relaxing or inspiring.								
I connected with others by visiting or speaking with a friend or family member.								
I rewarded myself with a massage, movie, small gift, or a pat on my own back for how well I got through the day.								
I delegated duties to relieve stress.								
I shared a hug with a loved one or animal friend.								

RESOURCES

Supplements and Other Products

Apex Energetics/Quintessential Healing, Inc.

www.annboroch.com ("Products" page) or call Apex at:

(800) 736-4381; (949) 251-0152 (international orders)

To order from Apex, you must call and set up a patient account with the number P2017; orders cannot be placed online.

Products: Adrenal abX, Candida abX, Cellular Recharge, Gabatone Active, Gallbladder abX, Gentle Drainage, Gluco abX, Glutathione Recycler, Liver abX, RepairVite (K-63, caramel flavor), Resvero Active, Serotone Active, Turmero Active

Bio-Design

(800) 822-6193 (say you were referred by Ann Boroch)

Products: Aloe Lite, Aloe 225

Emerson Ecologics

High-grade professional line of vitamins, supplements, and herbs

www.emersonecologics.com; (800) 654-4432

Tell customer service that you want to set up a patient account under Ann Boroch and give the code **Quint1** and **91604**.

Brands: BioPharma Scientific, Designs for Health, Douglas Laboratories, Gaia Herbs, Innate Response

General Ecology, Inc.

www.generalecology.com/products.php; 800-441-8166

Products: Water filtration systems, including portable system using structured matrix technology

Get Healthy Again

www.gethealthyagainstore.com; (800) 832-9755

Product: UltraImmune 9

Interceuticals, Inc.

www.betterwomannow.com; (888) 686-2698

Product: Better WOMAN

Invision International

www.silver100.com; (800) 454-8464

Products: Silver 100: colloidal silver spray, drops, and nasal spray

Koehler Co., USA

www.koehlerusa.com

(928) 541-1920 (say you were referred by Ann Boroch)

Product: Mynax

Landis Revin

www.landisrevin.com

(888) 908-7325 (ask for Mona Hoedel)

Either call and speak to Mona or follow these instructions to order online: Go to www.landisrevin.com. At the upper right-hand corner of the home page, click on "Healthcare Professionals." Click on the Trevinol Professional product you want and add to your cart. On the payment page, there's a place to enter a coupon code. To receive a discount, enter the coupon code for the amount of capsules you're ordering: the code for 90 caps is **Boroch90**; the code for 300 caps is **Boroch300**.

Product: Trevinol Professional

Long Life Unlimited

www.longlifeunlimited.com/category.sc?categoryId=69

(877) 433-3962

Product: Aclare Air purifier

Mendocino Medicinal

www.mendocinomedicinal.com; (707) 459-2101

Products: Tri-Kelp (sea cabbage, bull kelp, palm kelp)—iodine source to maintain healthy thyroid function and offset negative effects of radiation. Consume daily in a smoothie or with food. Also a supplier of topical compounds for pain and skin afflictions.

Metagenics

www.drann.meta-ehealth.com (register and order online)

Products: Benesom, Cenitol, High Concentrate EPA-DHA Liquid (lemon), Ultra Potent-C Powder

Mountain Rose Herbs

www.mountainroseherbs.com; (800) 879-3337

Products: Organic bulk herbs: dandelion root, hibiscus, red clover dried herb, pau d'arco, chamomile, peppermint

The Natural Bladder

www.thenaturalbladder.com; (800) 566-5522

Product: Bladder-Control

Pacific Botanicals

www.pacificbotanicals.com; (541) 479-7780

Products: Organic bulk herbs: dandelion root, hibiscus, red clover dried herb, pau d'arco, peppermint, chamomile

Ionic Researchers Association

www.annboroch.com (click on "Products" tab and scroll down the page, right-hand side)

Product: Ionic S.P.A. (footbath)

Vitamin Warehouses

These online warehouses sell vitamins, food, and natural body-care products at reduced prices.

www.vitacost.com

www.amazon.com

www.iherb.com

Brands: BioPharma Scientific, Biotics Research, Bob's Red Mill, Carlson, Christopher's, Douglas Laboratories, Essential Formulas, Enzymatic Therapy, Enzymedica, Gaia Herbs, Garden of Life, George's, HealthForce Nutritionals, Heel/BHI, Himalaya USA, Imperial Elixir, Jarrow Formulas, Life Extension, Lily of the Desert, Metagenics, Natural Factors, Natural Vitality, Nature's Way, Nordic Naturals, NutriBiotic, NutriCology/Allergy Research, Planetary Herbals, Priority One, Rainbow Light, ReNew Life, Solaray, Solgar, Source Naturals, Spectrum, Superior Source, Traditional Medicinals, Twin Labs, Vibrant Health, Vitacost, World Nutrition, Xymogen

Vollara

www.vollara.com

(800) 989-2299 (sign up under #315799)

Products: Air purifying and water systems

Waiora

www.mywaiora.com/740982

(866) 699-3467

Product: Natural Cellular Defense

Manufacturers and Suppliers
of Specialty Foods and Beverages

The majority of products I recommend can be ordered on amazon.com, vitacost.com, and iherb.com, or by going directly to the manufacturers' websites, including those listed below, if you cannot find them in your local health food store.

Awesome Foods

www.awesomefoods.com

Products: Raw breads and chips

Basiltops

www.basiltops.com

Products: Dairy-free spicy and non-spicy pestos

Bragg

www.bragg.com

Products: Unfermented, non-GMO soy sauce; kelp seasoning; and stevia-sweetened beverages

Coconut Secret

www.coconutsecret.com

Products: Raw Coconut Aminos, Raw Coconut Flour

DNA Life Bars

www.dnalifebars.com

Enter coupon code **boroch10** to save 10% or go to www.annboroch .com and order from the Products page.

Products: Protein squares and treats

Food for Life

www.foodforlife.com

Products: Brown rice tortillas, black rice tortillas

Go Raw

www.goraw.com

Products: Cereals, chips, crackers, nuts, and seeds

Julian Bakery

www.julianbakery.com

Products: Paleo Bread (almond or coconut)

Lydia's Organics

www.lydiasorganics.com

Products: Raw breads, cereals, chips, and crackers

Majestic Garlic

www.majesticgarlic.com/index.php

Products: Garlic spreads in various flavors

Mauk Family Farms

www.maukfamilyfarms.com

Products: Flax crackers and crusts

Nut Just a Cookie

www.nutjustacookie.com

Products: Nutty Nibbles cookies; choose sugar-free varieties

Rox Chox

www.roxchox.blogspot.com/p/all-about-rox-chox.html

Products: Organic chocolate treats sweetened with xylitol; made with raw cacao and coconut

Sami's Bakery

www.samisbakery.com

Products: Millet & Flax Bread (Wait at least 90 days to integrate any of their other millet and flax products because of added yeast; and even then eat only small amounts, as it may aggravate candida in some people's bodies and cause bloating. Make sure there is no sugar in the product.)

Sea Tangle Noodle Company

www.kelpnoodles.com/index.html

Products: Kelp noodles

Steve's PaleoGoods

www.stevespaleogoods.com

Products: Steve's Original Paleo Stix (grass-fed beef sticks)

Two Moms in the Raw

www.twomomsintheraw.com

Products: Flax crackers

Books on Candida and MS

Boroch, Ann. *The Candida Cure*. Quintessential Healing Publishing, Inc., 2012.

Crook, William G., MD. *The Yeast Connection: A Medical Breakthrough*. Vintage Books, 1986.

_____. *The Yeast Connection Handbook*. Square One Publishers, 2007.

_____. *Yeast Connection Success Stories: A Collection of Stories from People Who Are Winning the Battle Against Devastating Illness*. Square One Publishers, 2007.

Crook, William G., MD, with Elizabeth B. Crook and Hyla Cass. *The Yeast Connection and Women's Health*. Square One Publishers, 2007.

Graham, Judy. *Managing Multiple Sclerosis Naturally: A Self-Help Guide to Living with MS*. Healing Arts Press, 2010.

Kaufmann, Doug A. *The Fungus Link to Health Problems*. MediaTrition, 2010.

Perlmutter, David, MD. *BrainRecovery.com: Powerful Therapy for Challenging Brain Disorders*. Perlmutter Health Center, 2000.

_____. *Grain Brain: The Surprising Truth about Wheat, Carbs, and Sugar—Your Brain's Silent Killers*. Little, Brown and Company, 2013.

Perlmutter, David, MD, and Alberto Villoldo, PhD. *Power Up Your Brain*. Hay House, 2012.

Sawyer, Ann, and Judith Bachrach. *The MS Recovery Diet*. Avery Trade, 2007.

Swank, Roy L., MD, PhD, and Barbara B. Dugan. *The Multiple Sclerosis Diet Book.* Doubleday, 1987.

Trowbridge, John P., MD, and Morton Walker, DPM. *The Yeast Syndrome: How to Help Your Doctor Identify and Treat the Real Cause of Your Yeast-Related Illness.* Bantam Books, 1986.

Truss, C. Orian, MD, *The Missing Diagnosis.* Missing Diagnosis, Inc., 1985.

———. *The Missing Diagnosis II.* Missing Diagnosis, Inc., 2009.

Wahls, Terry L., MD. *Minding My Mitochondria: How I Overcame Secondary Progressive Multiple Sclerosis (MS) and Got Out of My Wheelchair,* 2nd ed. TZ Press, 2010.

Wahls, Terry L., MD, and Eve Adamson. *The Wahls Protocol: How I Beat Progressive MS Using Paleo Principles and Functional Medicine.* Avery, 2014.

Williams, Montel, and William Doyle. *Living Well: 21 Days to Transform Your Life, Supercharge Your Health, and Feel Spectacular.* NAL Trade, 2008.

Cookbooks

NOTE: Follow your "Foods to Eat" list, as there are differences in what some candida and allergy books allow and don't allow. You can also do an Internet search by typing in "candida recipes" and find many free recipes. Make sure to alter ingredients to match your "Foods to Eat" list.

Connolly, Pat, and Associates of the Price-Pottenger Nutrition Foundation. *The Candida Albicans Yeast-Free Cookbook: How Good Nutrition Can Help Fight the Epidemic of Yeast-Related Diseases.* McGraw-Hill, 2nd edition, 2000.

Crook, William G., MD, and Marge H. Jones, RN. *The Yeast Connection Cookbook: A Guide to Good Nutrition and Better Health.* Square One Publishers, 2007.

Greenberg, Ronald, MD, and Angela Nori. *Freedom from Allergy Cookbook.* Blue Poppy Press, 2000.

Jones, Marjorie H., RN. *The Allergy Self-Help Cookbook.* Rodale Books, 2001.

Martin, Jeanne Marie, and Zoltan P. Rona. *Complete Candida Yeast Guidebook: Everything You Need to Know About Prevention, Treatment & Diet*, rev. 2nd ed. Prima Health, 2000.

Semon, Bruce, MD, PhD, and Lori Kornblum. *Feast Without Yeast: 4 Stages to Better Health*. Wisconsin Institute of Nutrition, 1999.

Turner, Kristina. *The Self-Healing Cookbook: Whole Foods to Balance Body, Mind and Moods*. Earthtones Press, rev. ed., 2002.

Magazines on Nutrition and Health

Life Extension (monthly magazine, also a supplement company)
www.lifeextensionretail.com

Townsend Letter (monthly magazine)
www.townsendletter.com; (360) 385-6021

Well Being Journal (magazine published 6 times a year)
www.wellbeingjournal.com; (775) 887-1702

Natural Health and Advocacy Websites

These natural health newsletters and websites provide information on nutrition, supplements, advocacy, and natural solutions for healing.

www.anh-usa.org (Alliance for Natural Health)

www.livestrong.com

www.mercola.com

www.naturalcures.com

www.naturalnews.com

www.thenhf.com (The National Health Federation)

www.organicconsumers.org (Organic Consumers Association)

www.price-pottenger.org (Price-Pottenger Nutrition Foundation)

Books and Resources on Mind-Body Healing

Byrne, Rhonda. *The Secret* (DVD): a film that can help you change your life for the better. Prime Time Productions, 2006. See http://www .thesecret.tv/index.html.

Chopra, Deepak. *Quantum Healing: Exploring the Frontiers of Mind/Body Medicine*. Bantam, 1990.

Dawson, Jasmine Contor. *Aliens to Zebras*. Tao Song, 2005.

Dwoskin, Hale. *The Sedona Method: Your Key to Lasting Happiness, Success, Peace and Emotional Well-Being*. Sedona Press, 2003.

Emotional Freedom Technique, http://www.emofree.com. This therapeutic technique helps you to release fears, phobias, addictions, cravings, and fear-based and negative thoughts and emotions.

Hay, Louise L. *You Can Heal Your Life*. Hay House, 1999.

I Can Be Fearless app. This application helps in eliminating thoughts, feelings and actions that stop you from doing what you actually want to do. The process helps to remove old habits and patterns embedded in long-term memory that result in fear, worry, demotivation, grief, sorrow, loneliness, anger, and rejection.

Kasl, Charlotte. *If the Buddha Got Stuck: A Handbook for Change on a Spiritual Path*. Penguin Books, 2005.

Lipton, Bruce H. *The Biology of Belief: Unleashing the Power of Consciousness, Matter, & Miracles*. Hay House, 2008.

Maté, Gabor, MD. *When the Body Says No: Exploring the Stress-Disease Connection*. Wiley, 2011.

Myss, Caroline, PhD. *Anatomy of the Spirit*. Three Rivers Press, 1997.

Pert, Candace B. *Molecules of Emotion: The Science Behind Mind-Body Medicine*. Touchstone, 1997.

Siegel, Bernie S. *Love, Medicine and Miracles*. Random House, 1999.

Wilde, Stuart. *Infinite Self: 33 Steps to Reclaiming Your Inner Power*. Hay House, 1996.

Health Documentaries

The Business of Disease (2014)

Food, Inc. (2008)

Fat, Sick & Nearly Dead (2010)

Fast Food Nation (2006)

Food Matters (2008)

Fresh (2009)

The Future of Food (2004)

Genetic Roulette: The Gamble of Our Lives (2012)
King Corn: You Are What You Eat (2007)
A Delicate Balance: The Truth (2008)
Processed People (2009)
Unacceptable Levels (2012)

Laboratories

Diagnos-Techs
Salivary hormonal testing
www.diagnostechs.com
(206) 251-0596

Cyrex Laboratories
Multi-tissue antibody testing for autoimmune conditions, gluten intolerance, and cross-reactivity food sensitivities
www.cyrexlabs.com
(602) 759-1245

Direct Labs
www.directlabs.com
(800) 908-0000
Lab provides blood chemistry panels without needing a doctor's prescription, including the Apex 4 panel (a full blood chemistry panel with a vitamin D test)

Genova Diagnostics
Stool and blood testing for candida, parasites, and gluten intolerance
www.gdx.net
(800) 522-4762

Metametrix Clinical Laboratory
Metabolic, toxicant, and nutritional testing
www.metametrix.com
(800) 221-4640

NOTES

CHAPTER 1

1. William G. Crook, *The Yeast Connection: A Medical Breakthrough* (New York: Vintage Books, 1986).
2. Andrew Weil, *Spontaneous Healing: How to Discover and Enhance Your Body's Natural Ability to Maintain and Heal Itself* (New York: Ballantine Books, 1995), 308.

CHAPTER 2

1. Michael J. Goldberg, "Autism and the Immune Connection," http://www.neuroimmunedr.com/articles.html.
2. Christina M. Hull, Ryan M. Raisner, and Alexander D. Johnson, "Evidence for Mating of the 'Asexual' Yeast *Candida albicans* in a Mammalian Host," *Science* 289, no. 5477 (July 2000).
3. C. Orian Truss, *The Missing Diagnosis* (Birmingham, AL: The Missing Diagnosis, Inc., 1985).
4. David Perlmutter, *BrainRecovery.com: Powerful Therapy for Challenging Brain Disorders* (Naples, FL: Perlmutter Health Center, 2000).
5. David Perlmutter, "Fatigue in Multiple Sclerosis," *Townsend Letter for Doctors and Patients* 148 (1995): 48.
6. William G. Crook, *The Yeast Connection Handbook* (Jackson, TN: Professional Books, 1999).
7. J. P. Nolan, "Intestinal Endotoxins as Mediators of Hepatic Injury: An Idea Whose Time Has Come Again," *Hepatology* 10, no. 5 (November 1989): 887–91.
8. C. Orian Truss, *The Missing Diagnosis* (Birmingham, AL: The Missing Diagnosis, Inc., 1985).

CHAPTER 3

1. Keith W. Sehnert, Gary Jacobson, and Kip Sullivan, "Is Mercury Toxicity an Autoimmune Disorder?" *Townsend Letter for Doctors and Patients* 147 (1999): 134–37.
2. Donald H. Gilden, "Viruses and Multiple Sclerosis," *JAMA* 286 no. 24 (December 2001): 3127–29.
3. Miller et al., *British Medical Journal* 2 (1967): 210–13.

4. D. Geier and M. Geier, "Chronic Adverse Reactions Associated with Hepatitis B Vaccination," *The Annals of Pharmacotherapy* 36, no. 12 (2002): 1970–71.

Chapter 4

1. Kelly M. Adams et al., "Status of Nutrition Education in Medical Schools," *American Journal of Clinical Nutrition* 83, no. 4 (April 2006): 941S–944S, http://ajcn.nutrition.org/content/83/4/941S.full.

2. Interview with Gerald Ross, MD, "Toxic Brain Syndrome," *Mastering Food Allergies Newsletter* XI, no. 2 (March-April 1996).

3. Ann Louise Gittleman, *How to Stay Young and Healthy in a Toxic World* (Chicago: Keats Publishing, 1999).

4. Ray C. Wunderlich, Jr., and Dwight K. Kalita, *Candida Albicans: How to Fight an Exploding Epidemic of Yeast-Related Diseases* (New Canaan, CT: Keats Publishing, 1984).

5. Sharon Begley, "The End of Antibiotics," *Newsweek* 123, no. 13 (March 28, 1994): 48.

6. W. F. Nieuwenhuizen et al., "Is Candida Albicans a Trigger in the Onset of Coeliac Disease?" *Lancet* 361, no. 9375 (June 2003).

7. Marios Hadjivassiliou et al., "Gluten Sensitivity: From Gut to Brain," *Lancet Neurology* 9, no. 3 (March 2010): 318–30.

8. F. Batmanghelidj, *Your Body's Many Cries for Water* (Falls Church, VA: Global Health Solutions, 1995).

Chapter 5

1. M. Percival, *Functional Dietetics: The Core of Health Integration* (Ontario, Canada: Health Coach Systems International, 1995).

2. Jeffrey Bland, "Leaky Gut: A Common Problem with Food Allergies," interview by Marjorie Hunt Jones, RN, *Mastering Food Allergies Newsletter* VIII, no. 5 (September-October 1993).

3. Jeroen Visser et al., "Tight Junctions, Intestinal Permeability, and Autoimmunity: Celiac Disease and Type 1 Diabetes Paradigms," *Annals of the New York Academy of Sciences* 1165 (May 2009): 195–205.

4. N. Klotz and N. Ulrich, "Natural Benzodiazepines in Man," *Lancet* 335 (1990): 992.

Chapter 6

1. *Health Studies Collegium Information Handbook* (Reston, VA: Serammune Physicians Laboratories, 1992).

2. U.S. EPA Office of Toxic Substances, Stats from 1989 Toxic Release Inventory National Report.

3. W. Ott and J. Roberts, "Everyday Exposure to Toxic Pollutants," *Scientific American* 278 (February 1998): 86–91.
4. Interview with Gerald Ross, MD, "Toxic Brain Syndrome," *Mastering Food Allergies Newsletter* XI, no. 2 (March-April 1996).
5. See the documentary *Genetic Roulette: The Gamble of Our Lives* (download or order at http://geneticroulettemovie.com or http://www .amazon.com). Also see the mini-documentary *GMO Ticking Time Bomb* at http://www.naturalnews.com/037438_GMO_time_bomb_ Gary_Null.html.

CHAPTER 7

1. Shad Helmsetter, *What to Say When You Talk to Yourself* (New York: Pocket Books, 1986).
2. Bruce Lipton, *The Biology of Belief: Unleashing the Power of Consciousness, Matter, and Miracles* (Santa Rosa, CA: Mountain of Love/Elite Books, 2005): 132.
3. Elisabeth Kübler-Ross and David Kessler, *Life Lessons: Two Experts on Death and Dying Teach Us About the Mysteries of Life and Living* (New York: Scribner, 2000): 138–39.
4. Ed and Deb Shapiro, "Overcoming F.E.A.R.: False Evidence Appearing Real," Oprah.com, April 30, 2010, http://www.oprah.com/spirit/ Transform-Your-Fear-Into-Courage/2.
5. Gabor Maté, *When the Body Says No: Exploring the Stress-Disease Connection* (Hoboken, NJ: John Wiley & Sons, 2011; Alfred A. Knopf Canada, 2003): 20. Citations are to the Knopf edition.

CHAPTER 8

1. John Parks Trowbridge and Morton Walker, *The Yeast Syndrome* (New York: Bantam Books, 1986).
2. C. Orian Truss, *The Missing Diagnosis* (Birmingham, AL: The Missing Diagnosis, Inc., 1985).
3. John Parks Trowbridge and Morton Walker, *The Yeast Syndrome*.
4. Ibid.

CHAPTER 9

1. David Perlmutter, *BrainRecovery.com: Powerful Therapy for Challenging Brain Disorders*, (Naples, FL: Perlmutter Health Center, 2000).

CHAPTER 10

1. F. Batmanghelidj, *Your Body's Many Cries for Water* (Falls Church, VA: Global Health Solutions, 1995).

ABOUT THE AUTHOR

Ann Boroch is a certified nutritional consultant, naturopath, educator, author, and inspirational speaker. She specializes in allergies, autoimmune diseases, and gastrointestinal and endocrine

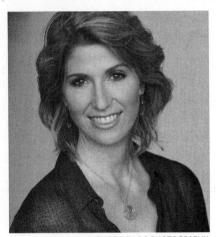

PHOTO BY OG PHOTOGRAPHY

disorders and is an expert on candida. Her successful practice in Los Angeles, California, has helped thousands of clients achieve optimum health.

Ann's passion is to help people realize that the body has an innate intelligence that allows it to heal itself—the key is to give it the right environment for a long enough period of time to remove inflammation and infection. She firmly believes that with choice and diligence, each of us has the power to overcome any challenge.

Ann has appeared on national radio and television, including a feature appearance on *The Montel Williams Show*, where she discussed healing multiple sclerosis.

For more information, contact:
 Website: www.annboroch.com
 Email: ann@annboroch.com
 Phone: (818) 763-8282